ANABOLIC MEN

THOR

by Christopher Walker and Ali Kuoppala

I

still remember the day…

It was another one of those awfully long Sundays when I had to go back to the military training facility I was serving at, 150 miles away from my hometown.

I plug in some music and prepare for a long bus ride into what will be few weeks of intense training…

…During these painfully boring bus trips that occur way too often, I read a lot – not books – but blog articles and studies about natural testosterone optimization.

On most of these trips, I endure the common half-assed blog posts about how to boost testosterone levels, the mounting pile of over-hyped rodent studies, and the horrible "testosterone boosting" training info that you can find on the depths of internet (you know what I mean, the usual "squats and deadlifts bro" type of articles).

Then I suddenly find something interesting.

An article by a guy named *Christopher Walker*. Not just any article, but a specific story about how he went from 11 ng/dL testosterone levels all the way to 1192 ng/dL in just 18 months, 100% naturally.

I finish the article thinking;

"This has to be the best article about testosterone optimization I've ever read."

Then I close the browser, drift into sleep, and completely forget about ever reading the article (no I don't have Alzheimers, I just had a lot of other things on my mind at the time, haha).

Time goes by, I get out of the army, and instead of going back to repairing cars, I start a blog about natural testosterone optimization (after all, the topic had been my passion for years, it was what I was truly interested in)...

...The website gains some traction, and eventually becomes a booming business, slowly building into an "authority" resource about the topic of natural hormone optimization.

Then I hear about this e-book called Testosterone I/O (now known as TestShock). I've heard that it's easily the best book about the subject available, but I'm skeptical about that at first.

I decide to read the book anyway.

During the preface I realize striking similarities between the book and the blog article I had read long time ago and forgotten...

"Wait. Is this the same guy?"

It is. The book is written by the same guy who went from 11 ng/dL to 1192ng/dL in 18 months, the same guy who had written that awesome story/blog article about his journey.

Chris Walker.

Suddenly my skeptic outlook towards the book flies out of the window. This guy know this topic. And I want to read the book.

Few hours and 262-pages later, I conclude in my mind;

"This has to be the best book about natural testosterone optimization I've ever read."

Immediately after finishing the book, I decide to contact Chris and start recommending his work to all my readers...

...Long story short, few years later and here I am writing the foreword to his new book, the very book you're reading:

THOR Program.

THOR is the finished version of something that the field of natural testosterone optimization lacked for years…

… A highly specific, evidence-based guide on EVERYTHING you need to know in order to maximize the training induced rise in testosterone levels, along with maximizing the long-term hormonal adaptations, eventually pushing your hormonal baseline higher and higher.

> **THOR is the finished version of something that the field of natural testosterone optimization lacked**

Reading TestShock – even after devouring thousands of studies about natural testosterone optimization for years before – was still an experience I haven't forgotten…

…All that new information, explained in a clear manner that only a true expert can come up with was something that you don't see everyday, especially within the topic of natural testosterone optimization…

…I expected nothing less from THOR, and once again Chris delivered the goods.

THOR is fresh. It's revolutionary. And it will once again change the game.

- Ali Kuoppala, AnabolicMen.com

"For your to-be-optimized testosterone levels".

Ali Kuoppala

Published by:

The Better Foundation, LLC

Acknowledgements

Special thanks are due to Ian Lenny for helping with content and ideas for this program, Rob Faigin for pioneering the concept of structuring your training with the purpose of hormonal health, Ray Peat, The Better Foundation team, Greg O'Gallagher (Kinobody.com) for all the discussions we've had around training philosophies for the past 5 years & for getting me to care about weight training in the first place, Jeremy Guymon for helping me expand a bigger vision for TS, Carter Good and Austin Floyd for being my THOR Protocol guinea pigs to test these methods, and to the AM Forum & Community members for your dedication to seeking truth and providing helpful information to one another and to all the past Anabolic Men success stories and the thousands of future ones that will come from this program.

Dedication

This program is dedicated specifically to every guy who reads its pages and is forever impacted with a renewed sense of control over their own destiny & health. Remember that you have complete control over your body and mind. You merely need to accept this, and you step into power beyond what you could ever imagine before.

Table Of Contents:

Chapter 1

The Optimal Way To Train As A Man

A man is not just a thing to be - it is also a way to be, a path to follow, and a walk to walk.

— *Jack Donovan, The Way Of Men*

H
ormonal optimization is the key to optimal health.

A radical idea. But a completely sound one. There is literally no better way to achieve optimal health than to train, eat, and live in a way that is completely aligned toward achieving hormonal homeostasis. *(This homeostasis – by its very nature – must always be pushed, however, as you will soon learn).*

This Truth is gender-apathetic. Men and women alike will benefit from awareness of this Truth. However, this book is written for men.

So all information herein is provided to advance your acceptance & application of this Truth, as a man. By the end of this program you will completely understand, without a shadow of a doubt, why it is either 1.) ineffective or 2.) counterproductive to your hormonal health to train your body in any other way.

Please read this program meticulously. The material I lay out over the course of this book is dense. However, I've attempted – to the best of my ability – to communicate it colloquially so anybody, regardless of educational background, can understand it easily.

The density of the material, coupled with a general societal lack of ability to think contextually (in this case, understand complex systems like the human body contextually) is the reason why so few people have ever laid out the argument you are about to read – and why so few people have ever asserted the one Truth I asserted above, in the first sentence of this book.

A necessary aside: I believe in universal truths and I am constantly in search of them.

THOR Training stands for Testosterone Hormonal Optimization Resistance Training.

In contemplating the potential name for this program, I was fortunate enough to think of this acronym, not only because it is cool (Thor is the Norse god of Thunder) but also because it is an easy-to-remember representation of this important training style, while emphasizing its utility.

Remember, optimal health equals optimal training + optimal lifestyle + optimal nutrition.

This program places a distinct and thorough emphasis on the "optimal training" variable in this equation. I also touch on optimal nutrition for this style of training in a chapter of this manual. But to read a much more comprehensive resource on achieving optimal health as a man, I recommend reading AnabolicMen.com where we have hundreds of free articles, a forum, and a Marketplace full of the best men's health solutions available from amazing brands.

That being said, I would like to emphasize three things in this introduction to the program:

- Program Devotion

- The Worldview For Dominance

- The Concept Of "Gym Dominance"

Program Devotion

While most training programs will implore you to "stick with it" to see results, I would like to appeal to your logical side instead of your emotional one. Asking you to *stick with it* implies that this is something I may or may not be forcing upon you. Something that would require constant "motivation" to achieve (ie. looking for energy from outside yourself to achieve internal progress). Something with an emotional motive, or association.

I personally think this is bullshit thinking.

Instead I will appeal to your logical side by – throughout this book – laying out the exact airtight argument for why THOR style training is the absolute only way you should be training your body. If I do my job properly, you will not need "motivation" to train this way. You won't need to "stick with it" in an effort to avoid "falling off the wagon."

If I do my job, by the time you understand the argument laid out here, you will be completely AWARE that this is the right way to train your body as a man. With that AWARENESS comes natural, effortless acceptance.

It requires no motivation whatsoever.

It is a natural acceptance of a Truth.

Also, when you become *aware*, you will naturally also understand that the most important aspect of this Truth is to operate based on the Principles at play, not necessarily the Details. The Details are only important in the context of the Principles, and therefore only need to be focused on after you understand the Principles. This type of thinking requires an acceptance of Balance – the opposite of neuroticism.

Neurotic thought is characterized by negative emotion and fear-driven avoidance behavior.

Neurotic men are more interested in avoiding an outcome than they are in producing results.

They are the type of people who experience conditions like "paralysis by analysis" and *orthorexia nervosa*, a psychological condition characterized by the development of an obsession with eating foods seen as "clean" and "healthy" to the point of being a detriment to the individual's health – typically to the tune of anxiety, social isolation, depression, severe malnutrition, micronutrient deficiencies, and loss of ability to eat naturally & appetite dysregulation.

A state of Balance will become not only desirable, but completely natural and effortless… because it is congruent with your acceptance of the Truth, and therefore inherently required to achieve the goal.

The Worldview For Dominance

My father is a retired US Marine Corps officer. He installed two core philosophies in my psyche from a young age:

1. You are entitled to nothing

2. Do something correctly, or don't do it at all

The US Marines are about as hardcore as warriors come. And they're 100% focused on Results derived from direct, swift, efficient action. So much so, in fact, that legend holds that at the Battle Of Belleau Wood in World War I, the German high command nicknamed them **Dogs From Hell**, *teufelshunde* (Devil Dogs), in response to the animalistic devotion to winning the battle.

To speak to #1 in the context of this program, you are not entitled to results. You must earn them through Work.

Which leads to #2, also in the context of this program: if you're not going to do this correctly, don't do it at all.

The Importance Of Actively Developing Your Worldview

You have a worldview. I have a worldview. We all have a worldview, whether you realize it or not.

Your worldview is the lens through which you see the world around you – and it means EVERYTHING to the life you end up living.

Most men *passively receive* their worldview throughout the course of their lives. They let other people impart their ideals upon them, then they receive (and subconsciously adopt) those as their own. Their lives usually manifest turmoil and mediocrity because of this passivity.

In short, and for lack of a better, more appropriate, more directly-applicable term: they get fucked.

To avoid this fate, you MUST actively build your worldview.

And the worldview of Dominance is a good one to develop.

This requires aligning your worldview to that of the development of authority in your pursuits. Authority implies mastery, control, power, status, and highest proficiency – all of which are inherently opposed to Entitlement. Which means you must **work** to become dominant.

When you accept that you need to Work to become Dominant, you naturally understand #2 from above – that there is no value at all in pursuing something unless you pursue it wholeheartedly because without this devotion you will never achieve the level of mastery required for authority.

And as a universal truth, this becomes an interesting line of thinking, because it is – as you will see when I lay out the physical & biological aspects of this program – completely paralleled to the way your body requires you to train for maximal hormonal output.

The Concept Of Gym Dominance

When you align your action toward a Dominant Worldview, it is only natural that you would see the gym as a training ground for developing Dominance.

You cannot truly have Authority in something without exerting that authority over it. Which means there must be a "subject" of that authority. In the case of the gym/weight room, this is the weight that you lift.

You will soon learn why progressive gains are *the only way* to truly optimize your hormones like Testosterone, Growth Hormone, Insulin, Cortisol, and DHT, among other androgens. But for now, I want you to understand that the gym should not be an "obligation" that you drag yourself to a couple times per week, nor will it be if you accept that the Truth in the first sentence of this chapter.

It is a symbolic arena for your development of authority over your physique & health via neuroendocrine response to progression.

For example, on machine lifts, while week-by-week progression is focused on increasing weight-lifted for the specific movement, the eventual intention becomes "full stack" lifting of the weight attached to that machine, which means that eventually you become able to out lift the level of resistance the machine can provide.

That all being said, as we wrap up the conclusion of this Introductory chapter, I want to make sure you fully understand the concepts I just outlined before we move forward into the biology. Without the understanding, the remainder of the book will be difficult to grasp on a Principle level (remember: this level of understanding is <u>required</u> before focusing on the details). Focusing on details before fully understanding principles will breed neurotic psychology patterns in men. Please avoid this. If you need to, re-read this chapter until these principles are all internalized.

" I want you to understand that the gym should not be an obligation that you drag yourself to a couple times per week.

Chapter 2

The Masculine Physique

Masculinity is not something that is given to you - but something you gain.

— Normal Mailer

Every man is hardwired to build more muscle in specific areas, and less muscle in other areas. Your muscle tissue – on the cellular level – is full of androgen receptors (ARs).

Certain muscle tissue groups have higher density of androgen receptors than other areas. This is naturally how our bodies exist, and once understood, can be used to our advantage in building a great looking physique with just the right amount of effort into optimizing the neuroendocrine response in muscle tissue with the highest density of androgen receptors.

With the proper training program designed to emphasize neuroendocrine response in these areas, the male body naturally looks how it is supposed to look – strong, powerful, imposing, with more muscle in the upper body concentrated in the shoulders, traps, upper chest, back and arms, and powerful legs without an unnatural amount of excess "limiting" mass.

Studies done on physical attractiveness in men are nothing new. Many people have discussed what creates "the perfect male physique" and how it differs from what the mainstream or even the fitness mainstream would have you believe.

What I want to do for a second is step back and take a look at some of the roots of male physical attractiveness and what shapes it.

While there are obviously many other things that factor into physical attractiveness, I want to focus on this as it is a key aspect of overall attractiveness and one that is much more appropriate for this manual.

Physical attractiveness in inexorably linked to a man's ability to fight and survive in the wild.

While this may be a surprising fact in our modern era, it has been shown time and time again in the research of anthropologists and evolutionary psychologists. One body of research done by by Aaron Sell, Liana S. E. Hone and Nicholas Pound found that attractiveness is largely related to apparent upper body strength.

Apparent upper body strength is seen as a combination of the shoulder to waist and waist to hip ratio. When researchers looked at the data, they found that a fairly tight set of measurements defined "the ultimate male physique". Basically the closer the waist to hip ratio was to 0.9 the better and the closer the shoulder to waist ratio to 1.6 the better.

The waist to hip ratio was taken by measuring at the narrowest point of the waist and the middle point of the hips. Similarly the shoulder to hip ratio was taken by measuring at the middle point of the shoulders and the narrowest point of the waist. The combination of these two factors provide a powerful insight into the automatic reaction people have to the different shape of a man's physique.

Waist to hip ratio and shoulder to waist ratio along with facial features, more masculine facial features being an indication of higher testosterone levels, allow people to accurately predict strength.

In human psychology, strength is used nearly interchangeably to predict fighting ability. So even though there are definitely people who look great but would never be able to hold their own if faced with any type of physical aggression, the association is nearly hardwired into the human psyche.

This dates back thousands of years when physical confrontation was a much more normal part of life. Anthropologist studying hunter gatherer societies have noted that some show death rates related to physical violence for males as high as 59%.

Statistics like that force a premium on apparent fighting ability as assessed through upper body strength.

The historical roots of human civilization dictate a specific interest in the fitness of a man's body via his assessed ability to survive the rigors of combat and the environment.

"The persistence of associations between upper-body strength and psychological and behavioral variables in modern men shows how powerful the selection pressures were: physically stronger men have been shown to feel more entitled to better outcomes."

The quote above comes from a study done on the roots of strength as a basis for male physical attractiveness.

The study looked at a number of factors associated with upper body musculature that caused it to be a primary attraction trigger. What they found was that the various utilities upper body musculature brought are the primary reason for its universal appeal.

Upper body musculature historically helped with throwing things at other people and animals, blocking things that were thrown at you. Crushing other things that you might want to crush as well as carrying things that need to be carried etc.

As you can see, there are a number of intuitive reasons why upper body musculature is a primary feature in the response other males and females have to the varying shapes of a man's physique.

It's important to note that the measurements discussed above represent a well proportioned male physique with noticeable muscle in the upper body.

This is a far cry from the bodybuilders and high level men's physique competitors you see in the magazines.

The measurements above also form a strong basis for my recommendation that you focus on training your lower body primarily for power. Training the lower body for hypertrophy would not allow you to conform to the standard mentioned above and would most certainly give you a lower body that appears less functional.

http://www.cep.ucsb.edu/grads/Sell/(2012)%20Importance%20of%20physical%20strength.pdf

Chapter 3

Understanding Androgen Receptors

Awake, Iron!

— Almogavares battle cry, showering sparks from their weapons

E very type of hormone has a specific type of receptor that it interacts with. The receptors themselves are usually a protein that is designed to receive the hormones as they travel through the bloodstream.

You can think of the receptor as a keyhole with the hormones being the keys. When the hormone floats through the bloodstream and reaches the muscle cells it fits into the receptor and unlocks a specific set of activities the cells are designed to be able to perform.

In the case of building muscle, the androgenic hormones fit into the receptors and begin the chain of events that lead to additional muscle tissue being created. Of course this process must happen in a massive amount of muscle cells for a noticeable amount of muscle tissue to be added.

The ultimate male physique relies heavily on the concentration of androgen receptors in the various muscle groups. The androgen receptors are the site on the muscle cells that interacts with the body's main androgenic hormones, testosterone and DHT. The interesting thing about these types of receptors is that the density of each type of receptor varies by muscle group.

Researchers have looked into the differences in androgen receptor concentration and how they interact with muscle growth and training. What they found is that androgen receptor concentrations in men are higher in the upper body than in the lower body. Specifically, the muscles of the chest, shoulders and trapezius have much higher androgen receptor concentrations than the muscles of the lower body.

What this means for guys looking to achieve the ultimate male physique is that changes in anabolic/androgenic hormone levels will cause a relatively larger change in the muscles of the upper body.

This is one of the reasons why steroid users usually show exaggerated levels of hypertrophy in the shoulders and traps. It also means that increasing your androgen levels through the methods described in the THOR Program will enhance your efforts to sculpt the ideal male physique.

In addition to studying the effects of anabolic hormones on androgen receptor density, researchers have looked into the effect resistance training has on androgen receptor density.

They do this by comparing the androgen receptor density in trained and untrained individuals. What they found is that androgen receptor density was higher in the trained individuals in the upper body muscles only. The density of these receptors did not increase in the untrained individuals to a statistically significant degree.

While the study did not show a significant increase in the density of receptors in the muscle cells, it said nothing about the amount of muscle tissue or the total number of androgen receptors. In this case we are talking about receptor density or number of receptors in a given area of muscle tissue.

The training increased the total amount of muscle tissue as well as the total number of receptors in both the upper and lower body while preferentially increasing the density of receptors in only the upper body musculature.

What this means is that when men perform resistance training workouts, the effects are more pronounced in the upper body.

More succinctly, men's bodies are designed for increased levels of muscle mass in the upper body.

Keep in mind, I am not saying you cannot have strength and power in the lower body. Men are capable of creating fantastically strong lower bodies capable of squatting massive numbers, sprinting at ridiculously high speeds and propelling their bodies onto even the highest box/plate stacks.

What I am saying is that men's lower bodies are not designed for high levels of muscular hypertrophy.

Just to reiterate, strength, power, and hypertrophy are all separate qualities.

While it is easier to have higher levels of strength with greater hypertrophy, it is not always necessary. In addition, power is not enhanced by high levels of hypertrophy. Therefore, you can still have a highly powerful and extremely strong lower body. You just don't want to have huge slabs of muscle piled all over your legs, glutes, and hamstrings.

Selective Hypertrophy to Take Advantage of Androgen Receptor Density

Another issue with high volume leg training is that it saps the central nervous system's ability to recover.

If you are training heavy squats and deadlifts on 2 separate days of a 3-5 day per week training program, you will have very little nervous system energy for training your upper body hard and then recovering.

As I mentioned above, training hard (especially upper body) is necessary to take full advantage of the body's ability to increase receptor density at the muscle cells. Only by maximizing the androgen receptor density can you take advantage of the increased circulating levels of anabolic hormones you should have following the THOR Program.

Instead of focusing too much on compound lower body resistance training exercises, you will focus on your big upper body lifts and your concentric focused neuromuscular training exercises like sprints and muscle ups. Unlike squats and deadlifts, sprints and muscle ups have a relatively small eccentric component.

The eccentric component of the exercise is the part where the muscles are elongating while under tension.

This is the phase of muscular action that is responsible for most of the physical damage to the muscle. It is a key component of hypertrophy training that sets the stage for the muscle to rebuild itself larger than before.

By minimizing this component of the exercise you are able to do a higher volume of high intensity work with a smaller amount of physical damage to the muscles.

This is the same reason that Olympic lifters drop their weights from overhead when performing a large amount of snatches or clean and jerks. They want to stimulate their nervous system maximally while minimizing the amount of muscular damage they incur during training.

Similar to the Olympic lifter's use of weight dropping we will use exercises that naturally limit the eccentric phase of muscle action for our neuromuscular training.

Sprints can stimulate the nervous system to a very high degree without causing the same amount of muscular damage as squats and deadlifts. Muscle ups allow you to get a high degree of nervous system stimulation with a relatively small amount of eccentric stress as well. Additionally, both exercises interfere minimally with the structural damage caused by your standard resistance training exercises.

Focusing your traditional resistance training exercises on your upper body musculature allows you to take advantage of your natural propensity to add muscle to the areas of the body with the highest density of androgen receptors.

Using exercises that de-emphasize the eccentric phase of muscle action for your neuromuscular exercises allows for the greatest impact on hormonal output while interfering minimally with structural recovery.

The emphasis on these two types of training, with a balanced amount of secondary types of exercise (stretching, lower body training, cardio), will create a strong, attractive and balanced physique.

The "Recomposition Of Mass" Principle

When you train your body in a way to maximize hormonal response in the areas where your body is most receptive to the hormonal increase (i.e. high AR density areas) your body will start to steadily undergo a "morphing" process, where you will gain muscle and lose fat naturally, and in a way that shapes your body.

This is the Recomposition Of Mass principle.

This is how you should be thinking about transforming your physique – not from "counting calories," "weight loss," or "rapid muscle gain." Not even "bulking" and "cutting."

Those things all foster an unhealthy, potentially neurotic, state of thinking. And they're not focused on what really matters – hormonal optimization.

Steady recomposition of mass with the right training will produce the masculine physique you're looking for.

Focus on the principles in this program, which are directed at certain training movements that will produce, over adequate time (i.e. you must be patient) the desired physique through the morphing process where the body is continually trained – through repeat exposure to the right stimuli – to require less body fat and more muscle mass (specifically, in the areas where it is required to adapt to the training load).

RESOURCES:

http://www.ncbi.nlm.nih.gov/pubmed/10664066
http://www.ncbi.nlm.nih.gov/pubmed/21070797

5 Simple Ways To Increase Androgen Receptor Density & Activity

Before androgens (testosterone or DHT) can make any changes in your body, they have to enter DNA. In order for them to actually get to the DNA, they have to be bound from blood circulation by androgen receptors in cells.

This happens naturally all day long around your body, but did you know that you can actually increase androgen receptor density, as well as enhance their activity at utilizing male hormones?

That's right, there are a handful of supplements, few specific training methods, meal timing pattern, and one pretty popular drink that have all been scientifically proven to increase androgen receptor density.

1. Intermittent Fasting

Intermittent fasting (IF) is gaining popularity like a rolling snowball. It's an eating pattern where you fast for majority of the day and consume all of your daily calories in a short eating window.

The most common method of this is the Lean Gains style where you fast for 16 hours and feast for 8 hours. This cycle repeats everyday.

There are many benefits to IF, things like improved insulin sensitivity, weight loss due to easier maintenance of the calorie deficit, and sharper cognitive functions…

…But did you know that insulin is not the only thing that your body becomes more responsive to after short-term fasting?

Androgen receptors seem to have the same effect towards testosterone and DHT after fasting, when you start eating. There are two studies which showcase this, one from Sweden which showed that fasting for 12-56 hours can increase the responsiveness to testosterone by up to 180%…

…And another one where the subjects actually did a 10-day water fast, then resumed eating and they were followed for 5 days as they consumed their normal meals, as you can see from the graph on right, their testosterone levels shot up like crazy and kept climbing for the 5-day post-fasting follow up.

The likely explanation here is that their bodies became more sensitive towards androgens during the ruthless 10 days of no calories whatsoever.

NOTE: No, I do not recommend anyone to do a 10-day water fast, shorter fasts like the 16:8 method should still do the trick, and those are what I recommend (more about those here).

2. Resistance Training

Resistance training is a reliable way to increase testosterone levels. Not only does it boost the production of the big-T, it also increases its utilization by up-regulating the activity and density of androgen receptors in muscle tissue.

Research has shown that trained men have significantly higher AR content in their muscles than non-trained individuals, and that different types of weight-lifting methods yield different degrees of AR activation.

Since androgen receptors are a factor in muscle protein synthesis, it's only logical that their density and activity increases after the body adapts to resistance training.

There are few "training rules" you should follow in order to maximize the androgen receptor increase, testosterone and DHT release, and of course, muscle & strength gains:

1   Activate large amounts of muscle mass, with proper form, and still remain somewhat "explosive".
2   Do it rather quickly in order to avoid increases in cortisol (which decreases AR content of muscles).
3   Progress with your lifts on a weekly basis, and rest accordingly to actually be able to do that.

Luckily, this is all explained in a detailed manner with actual exercise routines and periodization schemes here in the THOR Program.

3. Carnitine

Carnitine occurs naturally in meats and fish. In fact it might be one of the most hormonally useful compounds that vegans miss in their diets.

The simplified mechanism of action for how it can increase androgen receptors naturally is as follows:

Carnitine transports lipids (fat) into the cellular mitochondria to be used as energy -> androgen receptor (AR) activity within those same cells is increased.

These effects were shown in a study where 3-weeks of L-Carnitine L-Tartrate supplementation at 2g/day was able to significantly increase the amount of active androgen receptors in human subjects at rest.

The same researchers later replicated the study with exercising subjects to prove – this time with actual muscle biopsies – that in trained males, L-Carnitine L-Tartrate is even better at boosting AR content than what is seen at subjects who are sedentary.
Bottom line is that carnitine increases androgen receptors at rest and even more so after exercise. Using 1-2g/day of a similar tartrate for as used in the studies should do the trick.

4. Levodopa

L-DOPA (levodopa) is a naturally occurring amino acid found in high amounts in mucuna pruriens (velvet bean). It's a direct precursor to dopamine, can bypass the blood-brain barrier, and effectively raise serum dopamine levels.

In my previous article about mucuna pruriens, I linked few studies which showed how L-DOPA from mucuna pruriens was able to increase testosterone levels, raise dopamine, boost sperm health, enhance cognitive ability, and reduce prolactin levels…

…And as an icing to the cake, there's the fact that levodopa acts as a co-activator protein to the androgen receptors, effectively enhancing their activity in in-vitro studies (study, study).

Using 250-500mg's per day of quality M.Pruriens extract with standardized amount of L-DOPA should do the trick.

5. Caffeine

Caffeine, the principal alkaloid and active ingredient of coffee beans, is not only good at boosting your creativity and energy levels. The good stuff can also increase workout performance as well as increase androgen receptors and testosterone!

Studies on rodents have shown that chronic low-dose caffeine intake can increase testosterone levels, DHT levels, and androgen receptor (AR) expression.

The mechanism of action is that caffeine stimulates cAMP enzyme inside the cells that host the androgen receptor, and cAMP then stimulates another enzyme called protein kinase A (PKA), which then regulates the glycogen, sugar, and lipid metabolism inside the receptors, enhancing their activity at binding DHT and testosterone.

Caffeine activates AR with the same mechanism as forskolin does, by increasing intracellular cAMP levels. For better results, take your forskolin and caffeine in a fasted-state (insulin inhibits cAMP).

Conclusion on Androgen Receptors

There you go, five ways to maximize and increase androgen utilization at the receptor sites. To recap, here's your five-step natural AR optimization stack:

1   Drink some coffee in the morning in fasted-state
2   Pop few caps of forskolin, also in fasted-state
3   Crush a heavy workout (like this) in the evening (preferably still at fasted-state if u can).
4   Break the fast with a big post-workout meal and 1-2 grams of L-Carnitine L-Tartrate.
5   Before you go to sleep, consume 250-500mg's of mucuna pruriens extract.

Bonus: For poor guys who can't get the supplements; double the coffee, get the carnitine from red meat, and L-DOPA from fave-beans

Chapter 4

Testosterone 101

Deep in his heart, every man longs for a battle to fight, an adventure to live, and a beauty to rescue.

— John Eldredge, Wild At Heart

T estosterone is the principal male sex hormone. An androgen.

It is found in both males and females, and acts anabolically. While females naturally produce small amounts of testosterone, and have far greater sensitivity to the introduction of additional testosterone into their systems, males, clearly, are where testosterone is most prevalent (7-10+ times the natural amount of females), and in whom higher testosterone is most often desired.

It is secreted in the testicles of males, and ovaries of females, with small amounts also coming from the adrenal glands.

Androgens are steroid hormones, and can be produced naturally and synthetically. The presence of androgens in tissues that have androgen receptors promotes protein synthesis in those tissues, giving it anabolic influence.

Androgenic effects include much of what we consider to be human maturation, especially in sexual tissues/organs. For example, androgens heavily influence maturation of male secondary characteristics such as growth of the penis and scrotum, body hair, vocal sound depth, etc. Anabolic effects are characterized by things like muscle growth and strength, as well as bone maturation, increased density, and increased strength.

Testosterone gets to work, in both males and females, before we're even born and carries out its influence heavily first during the sexual differentiation process, then into infancy, prepuberty, puberty, adolescence, and adulthood.

T plays a role in many processes in the body, one of the more prominently known being spermatogenesis.

Without the presence of testosterone and/or the androgen receptor, spermatogenesis can't proceed past meiosis (ie. you can't produce sperm).

So now that we know where testosterone is produced, let's venture a guess at what may be the cause of low testosterone production.

There are two common culprits, and they're medically recognized as primary and secondary hypogonadism.

The first, primary hypogonadism, is caused by deficient testosterone production in the testis.

The second, secondary hypogonadism, is caused by hypothalamic-pituitary irregularities. They regulate your endocrine system. So for example, secondary hypogonadism can be caused when a piece of this puzzle isn't functioning properly. I'm of the opinion that these processes (primary + secondary hypogonadism) do not operate independently, as evidenced by the strong influence of the hypothalamus and pituitary gland on the gonads directly.

So in the end, it all comes back to brain health.

And therefore... gut health.

Your gut is your second brain. And you can directly influence its health with what you put into your body for nutrition.

Testosterone Deficiency

Ever wonder what it would feel like to be castrated?

No?

Male rat studies, give us a nice glimpse.

Castrated rats will cease ejaculating within a few weeks of "the big event" – even when testosterone has been missing from their bloodstream for almost that entire time (it generally disappears within a few hours of castration).

That reality gives us a glimpse of how powerful testosterone actually is in terms of pervasivity. Testosterone influences processes in the body for weeks after production has ceased. The hormone's effects take much longer to dissipate than the hormone itself.

When these castrated rats are treated again with exogenous (external/ foreign) testosterone, they resume normal behavior, as though never castrated. Take it away, and they cease ejaculating once again. And the cycle continues.

Testosterone, therefore, has what is known as an 'activational effect' on the body, with its presence promoting certain behaviors.

This example perfectly illustrates how something like hormone replacement therapy can have almost immediate effects on your system, but alas, they're transient, short lived, unless you continually apply the source back into the bloodstream.

Therefore, it's not a solution – just a bandaid.

So what does low testosterone look like? How do you know if you have low T without going to get it tested?

You can't know for sure without a formal test, but the following signs are good indicators of low testosterone:

1. Poor erectile function (strength of 'morning wood' is a decent way to measure)
2. Low libido
3. Fewer erections
4. Increased body fat and/or a difficult time losing it
5. Low energy
6. Low well-being (sometimes manifesting in depressive symptoms)
7. Low or reduced muscle mass

These are just some of the common symptoms, but they're broad, and could likely apply to many different causes, not necessarily just low testosterone. That's the main problem I have with the widespread use of generalized symptoms linked to specific ailments (you can go on WebMD and enter your symptoms and either have a.) the common cold or b.) brain cancer, for example).

However, if you have all of these problems, and have for a considerable amount of time, then there's a good chance your testosterone levels are not optimized.

A little more background on testosterone. You'll recall that testosterone is produced in the testis by cells called Leydig cells. The average plasma concentration of testosterone in human males typically falls between the range of 200 – 1000 ng/dl. In terms of timeline vs plasma concentrations over a lifetime, T levels rise sharply during adolescence, peak in a man's 20's, then begin a slow decline with age.

While its most potent and widely recognized effect on the human male body is its influence over the growth/development of sexual tissues, your testosterone level is also a good indicator of lean body mass (ie. muscle) potential, with the right stimuli.

Elevated testosterone levels will increase red blood cell production, bone density, sugar uptake into muscle tissue, muscle glycogen storage, and protein synthesis associated with muscular growth.

The Feedback Loop

The cascade of events leading to testosterone production begins in the hypothalamus with the release of GnRH (gonadotropin releasing hormone) which acts on the pituitary to produce two hormones: LH (luteinizing hormone) and FSH (follicle stimulating hormone). These are the gonadotropins.

Once in the bloodstream, LH makes its way to the testicles where it exerts its influence on the Leydig cells, triggering a series of events that turns cholesterol into testosterone.

As testosterone levels increase, LH production & transport slows.

A negative feedback loop.

The body and brain are communicating constantly in order to regulate important processes. This is one of countless feedback loops (there are many positive feedback loops as well) in the human body.

With this negative feedback loop, the brain can constantly keep hormone levels in check – in this case, testosterone, LH, FSH, and GnRH – under normal, healthy circumstances. When a problem arises anywhere on this pipeline, be it from a tumor, traumatic stressor, or summative build-up of small, unnoticeable toxic stress (super common) – not only is everything downstream affected, everything period is affected.

Because it's a loop.

Testosterone doesn't only linearly exert its influence back on the hypothalamus alone, it can also work directly back on the pituitary (essentially "skipping" a step) if your body is looking to quickly regulate gonadotropin release.

When this little system is working properly, everything's good. When something goes wrong down the line is when we run into noticeable issues).

FSH, the other gonadotropin, is chiefly responsible for stimulating (or regulating) production of sperm in the Leydig cells in the testis.

So at this point we understand that testosterone production is regulated by the brain, namely the hypothalamus and pituitary, via a handful of powerful hormones. And it's synthesized after a number of intermediate steps, from cholesterol in the Leydig cells. And this process is all tied together in a negative feedback loop.

Now it's produced. What happens next?

When testosterone is released into your bloodstream it is actually entering a molecular game of 'tag,' to put it metaphorically.

A carrier protein named SHBG, or Sex Hormone Binding Globulin, is released from the liver, and SHBG is 'it.'

SHBG's role is to regulate the level of freely circulating testosterone in your bloodstream. So when it binds a testosterone molecule, that testosterone cannot effectively enter and exert its influence on a cell (that's what she said).

So the more SHBG is in the bloodstream, the fewer testosterone molecules actually reach a cellular target.

This isn't inherently a bad thing, it's just the way things work. Another negative feedback loop meant to regulate your endocrine function.

However, now I hope you're beginning to realize the sheer amount of self-limiting processes that occur along the line in this cycle... and none of our testosterone has actually had an effect on anything yet!

With SHBG in this role, we now understand that testosterone levels and SHBG levels are inversely correlated: the more SHBG in your system, the lower amounts of free, active T.

Again, if something small is affecting ANYTHING along this pathway, you're likely going to experience an issue, manifesting itself as lower-than-optimal testosterone (and related hormone) levels.

For example, you may have very high levels of free, circulating testosterone, but with an imbalance in SHBG production, much of that free T won't reach a target.

Increasing Growth Hormone

Now let's talk about growth hormone.

First, what is it?

GH (or HGH, when referring to the collection of proteins in humans) is a peptide hormone secreted from the anterior pituitary and regulated by GHRH (Growth Hormone Releasing Hormone) and GHIH (Growth Hormone Inhibiting Hormone) – both secreted from the hypothalamus.

These two 'neurosecretory' hormones actually get released into the blood surrounding the pituitary and, in combination with physiological balance (heavily influenced by things like sleep, nutrition, exercise) they act upon the pituitary gland to initiate secretion of GH in a pulsatile manner.

Hopefully by now you're noticing a trend in how this works in terms of the HPG (Hypothalamus-Pituitary-Gonadal) axis. They also use pretty self-explanatory names for these hormones, which is nice.

Growth hormone is responsible for facilitating cellular growth, regeneration, and reproduction in humans and its effects are anabolic in nature. The bulk of your GH release occurs while you're asleep, with around half of it occurring between stages 3 and 4 NREM sleep. During the day it's been found to secrete in surges every 3 to 5 hours.

There are multiple ways to manipulate your GH secretion. Even just from what we've just learned we can easily see that by influencing the balance of GHRH to GHIH we'd be able to stimulate more GH secretion. Those neurosecretory hormones are also heavily influenced by the physiological downstream effects your body experiences from sleep, nutrition, and exercise – so those are some other things we'll explore.

Mostly because they're the easiest to control and measure.

Ghrelin is another lead. It was found to be a ligand for the growth hormone secretagogue receptor back in 2000, I believe... which in layman's terms means its presence can stimulate GH release.

A couple other natural GH release-stimulators are deep sleep, L-DOPA, fasting, and nicotinic acid (vitamin B3).

On the flip side, common GH inhibitors are 1. high circulating levels of GH itself or IGF-1 (due to the negative feedback loop) 2. glucocorticoids (ie. cortisol) 3. DHT.

Elevated (or even just normalized) levels of GH will make it much easier for you to build muscle (via increased ability to synthesize proteins), drop fat (via promotion of lypolysis), and spare glycogen (via reduced uptake of glucose in the liver).

So it's a good thing to have.

Anyways, now that we've introduced all that jazz, let's get into the training information. The big question: how should guys train if they want to naturally optimize their testosterone and GH production, and why?

Exactly How To Train For Optimal Hormonal Response (Short and Long-term)

Very recent study into the dual steroid (T and Cortisol) effects on training in elite athletes (as late as 2011), as opposed to older studies that often focused on untrained or moderately trained (with loose definitions of the word 'trained', varying from study to study) has, interestingly enough, opened up a ton of insight into this new paradigm for optimal endocrine response training.

In short, studying elite athletes gave us new insight into how average (untrained & moderately trained) individuals should train to optimize testosterone up-regulation.

The idea (in the following algorithm and program later in the book) is to use certain factors (workout design, nutrition, genetics, training status and type) to modify T and C concentrations and therefore influence resistance training performance and adaptive outcomes.

Changes in the concentrations of T and C can moderate or support neuromuscular (NM) performance through various short-term mechanisms such as 2nd messenger signaling, lipid/protein pathways, neuronal activity, behavior, cognition, motor system functioning, muscle properties, and energy metabolism.

A greater understanding over the recent years of T and C has led to suggestions that, beyond the more popular applications in morphological (ie. muscle size) and functional (ie. power and strength) enhancement, these hormones also exert heavy influence over NM functioning (ie. neuronal activity, intracellular signaling, and muscle force production), which means they contribute to the adaptive responses to training by regulating long term muscle performance via short term regulation of NM performance.

In short, we need to use NM training to influence long term muscle performance and optimize hormonal response to training.

It all comes back to my original philosophy of always addressing the roots of an issue as opposed to a symptomatic approach (and in life, operating on principles as opposed to stressing over details).

What is the neuromuscular system?

When I say NM system, I am referring to the peripheral nervous system (PNS in short). This consists of motor neuron units and innervated (stimulated to action) muscle fibers.

When looking to design a training program, we want to operate on the premise that acute elevations in endogenous hormones will increase the likelihood of receptor interactions, which will mediate long term adaptive responses.

Researchers are now shifting a lot of focus onto NM research in athletes because they're recognizing that neural factors may play a role beyond that of hormones, especially in early phase adaptations. However, the specific mechanisms for action still need to be examined as this is a relatively young (and ridiculously complex) field of study.

One thing that studying elite athletes made very clear to us is this: beginners may have a distinct advantage over highly trained individuals in terms of ability to elicit a workout-dependent testosterone and growth hormone response.

While elite athletes can generally elicit higher magnitude responses to their training, the stimulus needs to be far more specific.

For untrained or average individuals, the stimuli can be far reaching in variety and still elicit a high response, but they must operate on a set of known principles for the optimal response.

This initial testosterone response in untrained individuals is thought to occur mainly as an adaptive response of the NM system to support continual training under the new stimulus, which makes a lot of sense. Your muscles need to rapidly change to support your training, and the main way for them to do so (if you do the correct type of training) is to up-regulate androgen receptors with increased content and sensitivity.

So for the majority of guys reading this right now, even those who believe themselves to be highly trained (even if you are, it is probably in a very specific sport-related style) you will experience rapidly elevated workout-dependent testosterone levels with the correct training to assist muscular adaptation.

I will extrapolate this notion and speculate that even common weightlifters, crossfitters, and gym rats (ie. people with several years experience in resistance training) will find themselves noticeably untrained in this specific capacity when first embarking on this NM-style training according the algorithm I am going to propose.

Gymnasts and street workout guys will probably not have such a difficult time.

Endurance athletes, yes… it's going to be a big change.

(For example, several of my clients find they need at least one short nap per day along with a good nights' sleep to recover initially from the shift in training style during the first few weeks of the program, even though training sessions only run around 60 minutes in length – they adapt shortly thereafter).

To illustrate the advantage (I'm framing it as an advantage, but of course, it's all relative) that untrained individuals have over elite athletes when it comes to general T response to workouts (again, not magnitude, but reach and lack of specificity) I'll use an example that researchers found in elite 400m sprinters vs average individuals sprinting 400m.

In the elite 400m runners, every repetition decreased T levels post-sprint and increased LH levels (which, as you'll see in article 2, act as a precursor to stimulate T production). What this says is that they may have a decreased androgen receptor (AR) response to the training stimuli due to extensive training. Either that or an increase in glucocorticoid receptor (GR) sensitivity which would naturally suppress the T. I'd put money on the notion that it's a mix of both.

By comparison, the untrained sprinters saw a significant increase in T concentrations post-sprint with unchanged LH levels, indicating an increased AR sensitivity due to the new stimulus.

This indicates that it may be better for untrained individuals to hit harder fatigable bouts, but in low enough quantity to not elevate cortisol significantly, which introduces the idea of a training stimulus threshold.

A Formula For Optimal Testosterone Production via Training

Take what you just learned, and remember it. We're going to introduce a couple more concepts now, then mash them all together to formulate the perfect algorithm for training-induced T production.

Researchers have found that explosiveness encourages NM adaptations necessary to support the training demands (ie. indicating a long term adaptation), and that a training threshold very likely exists.

We want to up-regulate AR content in fast glycolytic muscle tissue (as opposed to slow oxidative tissue).

Resistance training is unanimously agreed upon as a potent stimulus for testosterone production and muscle growth, but the specific type is either not discussed or not agreed upon. What we do know is that resistance training promotes an increase in both AR mRNA (ie. gene transcription) and protein content and T concentrations.

So combining both of these ideas, we can come to the conclusion that explosive resistance training is the optimal form of stimulus – as long as it is performed under the performance threshold (so as to continually promote AR up-regulation without compromising due to cortisol/stress-related suppression).

But that's not the entire picture. It's also not entirely different from what the pop-fitness media promotes (though rarely practices).

One more key element to the equation is often overlooked.

And that's the idea of workload and its relationship to muscle volume activation (MVA) relative to intensity.

It has been demonstrated that the magnitude of the hormonal response to training is proportional to the size of the muscle volume activated. This is why we hear the old paradigm of "squat, squat, squat" to increase testosterone. Big leg muscles = more muscle tissue activated.

However, this MVA-dependent hormonal response is relative to the intensity of the movement performed.

Squatting high reps for hypertrophy training may stimulate GH and T production, but I'd argue that it won't be optimal because the intensity is not high enough, it is just drawn out over more reps. On the flip side, low rep squatting implies higher intensity, but allows for less total work done on the muscle.

Work, as a mechanical construct in physics, was originally defined by French mathematician Gaspard-Gustave Coriolis as "weight lifted through a height." The main equation you see everywhere is:

$$W = Fd$$

Where W is work, F is the magnitude of the force and d is displacement.

Researchers have found that, in terms of GH response, high amounts of work done – that is, high amounts of force related to the weight displaced – generated a significantly higher hormonal response to training than low work done.

So let's recap, and combine all of the knowledge up to this point in the article in order to formulate the idea of an optimal T-response-oriented training paradigm.

High work load, with a high proportion of muscle volume activated relative to intensity of the stimulus on said muscle volume, which should be performed via explosive resistance training done under a performance threshold (ie. self-limiting) = optimal.

Expressed algorithmically, it would look something like this in its simplest form…

W (MVA * i) < Stress Threshold

Where W is work (Fd), MVA is muscle volume activation, and i is intensity.

The stress threshold is defined as the point after which negative adaptations occur in terms of GR up-regulation and the subsequent increased sensitivity to stress-hormones, which are known to suppress androgen production.

So in short, we need to use this style of training, and walk the line under the stress threshold.

This is achieved best through explosive resistance and optimized by activating the most muscle possible over maximal displacement (at explosive intensity) while remaining just beneath the threshold.

I believe that in order to keep our training beneath the threshold, calisthenics becomes an increasingly attractive form of training due to its self-limiting nature and relationship with gravity (ie. if you can't do another muscle-up, you can't just subtract weight from your body as you could with a barbell in order to get additional reps or sets into the workout session).

This is based on the idea that in the 5-8 rep range you are able to perform an explosive set with high force and displace enough weight to keep total work high, but relative stress low. Much higher than 8 reps at the correct intensity will, I think, negatively affect your performance threshold, and any lower than 3 reps will compromise the intensity of the movement.

This is also why I advocate "enough rest between sets to recover just enough to perform another intense, slightly sub-maximal set" – no more, and no less. This will vary based on the individual but will probably fall in the 1-3 minute range based on the movement and the training level of the individual. 60 seconds rest appears to be optimal for GH output during a session.

RESOURCES:

Powers M (2005). "Performance-Enhancing Drugs". In Leaver-Dunn D, Houglum J, Harrelson GL. *Principles of Pharmacology for Athletic Trainers*. Slack Incorporated. pp. 331–332. ISBN 1-55642-594-5.Wren AM, Small CJ, Ward HL, Murphy KG, Dakin CL, Taheri S, Kennedy AR, Roberts GH, Morgan DG, Ghatei MA, Bloom SR (November 2000). "The novel hypothalamic peptide ghrelin stimulates food intake and growth hormone secretion". *Endocrinology* **141** (11): 4325–8. doi:10.1210/en. 141.11.4325.PMID 11089570.

Quabbe HJ, Luyckx AS, L'age M, Schwarz C (August 1983). "Growth hormone, cortisol, and glucagon concentrations during plasma free fatty acid depression: different effects of nicotinic acid and an adenosine derivative (BM 11.189)". *J. Clin. Endocrinol. Metab.* **57**(2): 410–4. PMID 6345570.

Nørrelund H (April 2005). "The metabolic role of growth hormone in humans with particular reference to fasting". *Growth Horm. IGF Res.* **15** (2): 95–122.doi:10.1016/j.ghir.2005.02.005. PMID 15809014.

Low LC (1991). "Growth hormone-releasing hormone: clinical studies and therapeutic aspects".*Neuroendocrinology*. 53 Suppl 1: 37–40.PMID 1901390.

Allen DB (September 1996). "Growth suppression by glucocorticoid therapy". *Endocrinol. Metab. Clin. North Am.* **25** (3):

Chapter 5

What Is THOR Training?

If you want something you've never had, you must be willing to do something you've never done.

— Thomas Jefferson

Like I mentioned earlier, THOR Training stands for Testosterone Hormonal Optimization Resistance Training.

This style of training places paramount emphasis on inducing hormonal response in muscle tissue that is especially receptive to these hormones, leading to more power development, a natural increase in muscle tissue (size & density), more androgen receptors available, and increasingly efficient neuromuscular pathways.

It is important to understand that every choice you make with your diet, training, and lifestyle – every single day – either impacts your hormones beneficially or negatively, so aligning your actions with positive progression in improving your insulin, cortisol, testosterone, and growth hormone balance over time will yield all the health & physique benefits you're seeking.

If you're not training correctly, you are either <u>ineffective</u> or <u>counterproductive</u>.

So what is the best way to train your body to trigger consistent hormonal output of testosterone and growth hormone?

Answer: You must train in the way that forces your body to adapt to the stimuli.

The only way to force your body to adapt is to push the boundaries of what you are currently capable of doing, consistently – week after week.

Think about it: your body is an amazing system that can adapt to just about any situation, with enough time. The way the body adapts is via hormones. When placed under (positive or negative) stress, your body will release certain hormones that trigger downstream responses from many metabolic processes.

The human body is constantly seeking a state of homeostasis (balance).

When a stressor is introduced that forces it to adapt, it will release hormones that trigger these processes in its "drive to survive" and eventually reach homeostasis once again.

Basically, your body is always seeking a "comfort zone." So when you push it outside of its comfort zone, and when you establish that this progression is not a temporary stress (i.e. you force it to adapt) your body will naturally begin establishing this as the "new normal."

You must train in a way that harnesses this progressive development (forcing adaptive change). This is the ONLY way to trigger significant, consistent neuroendocrine response.

This is best done through development of Power (I will discuss specifics later).

All training must be focused on this progression. Your body will only respond with positive hormonal adaptations in response to physical progression. You must continually force your body to do what it currently is not capable of doing… but soon will be.

Hormonal response to training stimuli only happens when the body needs to adapt, therefore you must push yourself to adapt to increasingly difficult stimuli.

The chart below perfectly illustrates this concept.

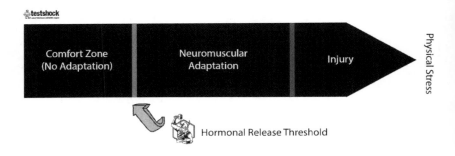

The comfort zone should be constantly changing. Right now, your comfort zone is where no adaptation will occur. It is your "normal." If you train in this zone, you will be either 1.) ineffective at inducing hormonal response or 2.) counterproductive, creating a worse hormonal environment than before.

Training above the threshold line, you force neuromuscular adaptation by triggering hormonal release. Your body will flood the bloodstream with free testosterone and growth hormone to increase binding to ARs, as well as increase overall amount of ARs available for binding (especially in the upper body), facilitating the necessary metabolic processes to support the positive stress stimuli. Remember, your body will do everything it can to create a "new normal" for itself. Use this to your advantage.

In the same way you can force progression via positive hormonal adaptation, you can also allow regression by doing the wrong types of training, which is counterproductive.

This counterproductive training that allows regression, essentially taking steps backward and hurting your health, is training that introduces negative stress on your system, forcing your body to chronically elevate cortisol (stress hormone) over time. I will get into more details soon, with regards to what types of training do this. You must avoid these types of training like the plague. They will only damage your health.

Remember, there is no such thing as a free lunch.

You MUST compel this adaptation.

This is NOT comfortable training. Embrace the discomfort, because discomfort is your new normal. If you are not in a constant state of discomfort with respects to the training stimuli you introduce, you are not improving. Your body will adapt, find homeostasis, and will find no need to release additional androgens. If you want high natural testosterone levels, and you don't want to waste your time spent in the weight room, then you need to constantly push the threshold.

Do not gravitate towards movements in your training that you find least intolerable and most enjoyable (until you begin finding that enjoyment in the midst of the discomfort ;), rather understand that your training effort is entirely based around forcing adaptation, and benefitting from the subsequent hormonal response.

This inherently requires discomfort, and literally defines the types of neuromuscular training movements that adhere to the Testosterone Work Principle.

Testosterone Work Principle: "Do as much Work on as much muscle tissue as possible in as short amount of time as possible while staying under the negative stress threshold."

Understanding all of this means that you also acknowledge the requirement for complete devotion to the protocol. You cannot – on THOR – supplement this training with additional training, or you will compromise everything and greatly increase your chance of injury by pushing your body over the negative stress threshold.

Limited Local Failure & Self–Limiting Training

To force neuromuscular adaptation, you must constantly cycle between Limited Local Failure (LLF) and recovery.

LLF is the top-end of the amount of work you can do on the muscle before it fails (in our case, at a given rep range – which means LLF is not 1 rep max 1RM).

For the sake of this program, this means 100% effort.

To leave the "comfort zone" and move through the threshold to induce a neuroendocrine adaptation response, this 100% effort is required. However, in the context of THOR training, the program is designed so that this 100% LLF effort is recoverable within 60-120 seconds back to near-baseline (we establish this by sticking to a specific rep range for lifts).

You must produce LLF or you are only asking your body to do that which it is already capable of. If it is readily capable of performing that task, then there is zero impetus for adaptation.

Contrast this with what is known as Systemic Failure.

Systemic Failure is characterized by the inability to recover quickly, crossing the negative stress threshold where cortisol release becomes counterproductive and impairs progress, rather than stimulating it (like LLF).

Common systemic failure training includes any style of weight or endurance/conditioning training that is characterized by high intensity over extended periods of time (usually includes rapid of loss of proper form on movements). People who induce systemic failure usually puke, or feel intense nausea during or after training.

Systemic failure can also occur if the individual trains near the negative stress threshold (not necessarily crossing it) too often, with little or no focus on adequate recovery between sessions. Burnout is typically the eventual result.

It is important to understand that positive stress is necessary to force progression. However, a threshold exists where stress becomes counterproductive to the point of impairing progress.

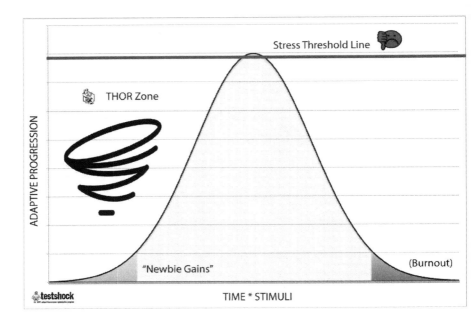

The 100% effort involved in Limited Local Failure is necessary because it takes you to the stress threshold but you don't cross it, because you physically cannot. Which means you maximize positive hormonal benefit without inducing any negative response.

This is the nature of self-limiting training.

Self-Limiting training is training that focuses on movements that inherently "self limit" by not allowing you to cross the negative threshold. For example, pull-ups... if you can only do 10 pull-ups, that means you cannot do 11. If you jump up and do your maximal effort of 10 pull-ups, then drop down, and I tell you to jump up and do another one... you cannot physically do another one, no matter how hard you try.

Pull-ups, in this sense, are self-limiting. You cannot push yourself over the negative threshold with pull-ups.

By utilizing a host of self-limiting movements in your training regimen, you will never cross the negative threshold, but you will have the ability to maximize your effort in the adaptation zone.

I like to think of THOR training as "Antifragility Training" – to adopt the term coined by Nassim Taleb.

In his book Antifragile, he defines it as the following: "Some things benefit from shocks; they thrive and grow when exposed to volatility, randomness, disorder, and stressors and love adventure, risk, and uncertainty. Yet, in spite of the ubiquity of the phenomenon, there is no word for the exact opposite of fragile. Let us call it antifragile. Antifragility is beyond resilience or robustness. The resilient resists shocks and stays the same; the antifragile gets better."

Build your training in a way that you benefit from stress, using it to force adaptation, and you will reap the hormonal rewards.

The basic idea behind programming exercises on the THOR program is going to focus on a few big compound lifts that you can progress on over time, while adding in assistance exercises to balance out your physique and keep the main lifts progressing.

If you had to sum the training principles up in one sentence that would pretty much be it.

If you wanted to get into more detail you could describe things like exercise rotation, sets and reps and specialty exercises for breaking through plateaus.

Specialty Exercises

First off I will describe the specialty exercises. Basically there are a number of specialized exercises that have been developed by strength athletes over the years to bridge the gap between the primary lifts and the isolation exercises used to train the muscle involved in those lifts.

A good example is the bent arm lateral raise.

This is an exercise that occupies the middle group between the compound shoulder press and the lateral raise. Unlike the press, it does not heavily recruit the triceps or trapezius.

What this lift does do is allow the trainee to utilize much heavier weights as well as momentum to overload the side delt.

This is unlike the straight arm lateral raise that is more conventionally used as an isolation exercise. The traditional straight arm raise can be use to great effect in the higher rep ranges, but presents some problems when trying to use heavier weights.

First, it can be limited by the trainees ability to stabilize the elbow joint during full extension. This version of the exercise heavily taxes the biceps and triceps as well as other muscles involved in elbow stabilization.

The other problem is that this version of the lateral raise does not allow the trainee to use momentum which prevents overloading the exercise through the negative portion of the rep.

By simply bending the arm you transform the exercise into a semi-compound movement where you are able to utilize torque generated at the hip to assist in moving a heavier weight than you otherwise would.

This allows you to overload the side delt through the negative portion of the rep and provides a novel stimulus to the shoulders.

How Body Part Sections are Laid Out

In each body part section I am going to first outline a list of the most effective multi-joint compound lifts. These are going to be your "checkpoint" lifts you will use to measure overall progress and gains in relative strength. I will then list all of the isolation exercises you can use to shore up any weaknesses and balance out the body.

Finally, I will go over all of the specialty exercises that can be used in instances where a plateau has been reached. This exercises are not ones that you necessarily have to use, but can be used if you are having difficulty breaking through a plateau or fill that your body would benefit from a specific stimulus.

Exercise Rotation

Exercise rotation is a widely used technique to maintain progress after an initial plateau. Exercise rotation, as the name implies, has to do with swapping out an exercise for another similar exercise when a plateau has been reached or in anticipation of a plateau.

The tricky part is knowing which exercise to rotate to and knowing where to start in terms of loading when switching to another exercise.

The first part of the equation is knowing when to use exercise rotation and knowing when to switch up your exercises. Basically you will want to start using exercise rotation when you have a plateau that you have tried to get past twice and are not able to continue progress.

So, if you are upping the weight consistently on standing shoulder press and you find yourself unable to up the weight during two consecutive sessions it would be time to start thinking about exercise rotation.

In this instance you might be rotating to seated dumbbell shoulder press, machine shoulder press or seated barbell shoulder press.

In order to decide what weight to use you would need to look into your training log. Simply find what weight you stalled out at during your last progression on the exercise you have rotated to.

Alternatively, if this is your first time using the exercise you will need to play it by ear and feel your way to a working weight during your warm up sets. Keep in mind that you should be warming up to a working set weight that allows you to work in the same rep range as you were using when you stalled.

So in the above example let's say you stalled in the 4-8 rep range on standing shoulder press and rotated to seated dumbbell press, you would then warm up to a working weight that would allow you to once again start to work in that rep range.

Progression Systems

There are a number of different systems that have been used to track progression for each exercise. The important thing to keep in mind is that nearly any system of progression will work if used consistently.

The other thing to keep in mind is that different progression systems cause different changes to the physiology of the body.

Nothing revolutionary there, but it is something many people do not consider. For example standard pyramid training where the weight is increased and the reps are decreased can work. However, it causes changes to the muscle tissue that may not be in line with what you need.

For example, standard pyramid training, as described above, used with short rest periods is an excellent system for causing sarcoplasmic hypertrophy.

That is, changes to the muscle tissue that are primarily metabolic and allow the muscles to perform a higher density of work. While this type of change is important and can provide an increase in muscle size, it cannot drive long term gains to the extent that increased maximal strength can.

Maximal strength has to do with a change in the ability of the nervous system to fire the muscle tissue as well as the contractile strength of the muscles themselves. We are looking for both of those adaptations, with the second one, changes in the contractile ability of the muscle driving changes in the appearance of the physique.

For this type of progress I would suggest a system of progression that is focused around strength gain.

For this reason I recommend starting with reverse pyramid training as it places a premium on continued increase in the contractile strength of the muscle.

RPT

Most people reading this will be familiar with reverse pyramid training. It is, as the name implies, a reversal of standard pyramid training where the weight is increased and the reps are decreased.

In this type of training you first warm up and then start you first work set with your heaviest weight. After your first work set you reduce the weight 5-15% on each consecutive set.

For example, using a 10% reduction, you might start a set with 300lbs, reduce your weight to 270 lbs for your second set and then to 240 lbs for your third set. In this way you utilize the heaviest weight when your nervous system and muscles are fresh and shift the focus toward volume, as a secondary concern, after your higher intensity sets are complete.

This allows you to gain many of the benefits of slightly higher volume work without ruining the effectiveness of the higher intensity sets. Keep in mind that this type of set/rep system is most appropriate for your compound lifts where heavy weights can be used.

For this type of set/rep scheme to work you should have a specific amount of reps you are trying to get before you increase the weight. Using the example above, you might want to increase the weight when you are able to get 4 reps at 300lbs, 5 reps at 270 lbs and then 6 reps at 240 lbs. Depending on how advanced you are you could increase all set's weight, 2 of the 3 set's weight or only one of the 3 sets weight. So for an advanced lifter you might only increase the last sets weight.

You would then use 300lbs, 270lbs and 245lbs for your three sets.

If you are able to once again get all 4, 5 and 6 reps you would increase the second set. You would then use 300lbs, 275lbs and 245lbs.

If you were once again able to get all 4, 5 and 6 reps you would once again increase the weight to 305lbs, 275lbs and 245lbs.

At this point all sets would have increased by 5 lbs and you would be starting the progression over aiming to get all of the prescribed amount of reps for your sets.

In reverse pyramid training you will generally be able to get an extra 1-2 reps for each 10% drop in weight on the bar. So in the above example if you got 4 reps with 300lbs, a 10% reduction to 270lbs should allow you to get 5-6 reps.

The next 10% reduction in weight would then allow you to get 6-8 reps etc…

You will only know from experience how many extra reps you are able to get with subsequent drops in weight. Due to differences in nervous system firing, muscle and bone lengths and insertion points some people may have widely varying results. Simply use the 1-2 extra reps with each additional set as a guideline.

As with everything in the THOR program, this is simply a template to get you started. The higher level results will come to those who apply critical thinking to the ideas I have laid out an experiment with their body in the gym.

In that "critical thinking" vein of thought, I also recommend you listen to your body. When push comes to shove, the most important set in this reverse pyramid style lifting progression is the first set of 5. This is where you must make your consistent progress.

If you find that adhering to a strict "drop" percentage for the 6, 8 sets after the 5 set is actually applying excess stress to your muscles in being too much work done, then I advise a larger drop in weight for those sets, so long as the 5 set is never compromised and is always progressing higher and higher in weight.

Straight Sets

Straight sets are an amazing companion to reverse pyramid training.

They work best with isolation exercises that are meant to shore up weaknesses and keep the main lifts you will be using RPT on progressing.

For straight sets you simple have a range of reps you are shooting for as well as a number of sets you will be performing. Say for example reverse lateral raises are going to be used for 3 sets totaling 8-12 reps each.

You simply start your first workout with a conservative weight you know you will be able to get all 8-12 reps in for each of the 3 sets. Let's say you use 10lb dumbbells and get 12,11,9 reps. Then on your next workout you once again use 10lb dumbbells and get 12,12,12 reps. you would then choose the next set of heavier dumbbells at your next workout, probably 15s, and start at the bottom of the rep range for 8,8,8 reps for your three sets.

This is a great system that allows you to keep progression on isolation exercises or secondary lifts with as little as one additional rep in any of the three sets.

Again, the two systems of progression are a guideline.

Many other systems will work if used consistently.

I would suggest sticking with these two until you have seen some success. If you do decide to use a different system of progression, keep in mind that it will only work if you stick to it and do not start to mix and match systems.

Sets and Reps and Rest

There are a bunch of different ways that you can alter your sets and reps for your workouts. I am going to go ahead and give a blanket recommendation as a starting point.

Keep in mind I am explicitly giving this as a starting point and in no way a concrete recommendation that cannot be violated. 2-4 sets for your main lifts in a rep range of 5-8.

Using RPT for your main lifts for 2-4 sets with a starting weight that allows you to get 5 reps is a great starting point. Depending on how taxing the exercise is utilize 3-4 minutes of rest.

For your assistance exercises utilize 2-4 sets as well with a weight that allows you to get 6-12 reps. Depending on how taxing the exercise is use 1-3 minutes of rest.

The above recommendations allow a nearly infinite combination of exercise set and rest protocols within a relatively tight set of recommendations. Though I have only given 2 system of progression, 2 sets of potential rest period lengths and 2 rep ranges, you should have enough flexibility to sets up programs for the rest of your life.

A question I get asked a lot is how many sets.

There are 2 ways I look at this. If you are on the lower end of your calories, keeping your time in the gym as short as possible will benefit you more than any additional training.

In this case do the minimum amount possible to maintain your physique or make limited gains while you cut. If on the other hand you are at maintenance or above maintenance calories, emphasize the exercises you want to progress the most on.

One caveat to emphasizing exercises is that you cannot emphasize everything. This is an idea that took me nearly a decade to realize.

Though it is tempting to include every productive exercise there is, the more you include of one, the more you dilute the effectiveness of the other.

That is definitely an idea you need to get in your head. Each additional exercise you add on is directly contributing to the diminished effectiveness of all other exercises in your program.

Exercise Selection

For the main "checkpoint" lift exercises in your program choose 1-2 for each workout. For the secondary and isolation exercises choose 2-4 for each of your workouts.

For your specialty exercises choose 0-1 for each of your workouts depending on whether or not you have a specific plateau or emphasis you are trying to focus on.

You do not want to make specialty exercise the core of your program as their continued use indicates a more fundamental error in your programming. In this case you most likely need to rethink your sets, reps, rest periods or exercise selection.

Please see the Protocol chapter for the recommended workout week.

Body Part Exercise Selection

In this section I am going to break down what I feel are some of the best exercises for the various muscle groups.

As mentioned above I am going to break the different exercises down into ones that would be best for your main movements, accessory exercises and specialty exercises used to break through plateaus.

Shoulders:

"Checkpoint Lifts"
Seated Barbell Shoulder press
Standing Barbell Shoulder press
Seated Dumbbell Press
Machine Shoulder Press

"Assistance Lifts"
Seated Dumbbell Lateral Raise
Seated Dumbbell Front Raise
Incline Bench Chest Supported
Dumbbell Rear Lateral Raise
Standing Dumbbell Lateral
Raise

Bent Over Reverse Lateral
Raise
Cable Lateral Raise
Cable Front Raise
Cable Rear Lateral Raise
Cable Rear Lateral Raise
"Specialty Exercises"
Barbell Seated Behind The
Neck Shoulder Press
Barbell Standing Behind the
Neck
Bent Arm Lateral Raise
Cuban Press

Chest:

"Checkpoint Lifts"
Bench Press
Incline Bench Press
Dumbbell Bench Press
Dumbbell Incline Bench Press
Weighted Dip
Machine Chest Press

"Assistance Lifts"
Flat Dumbbell Fly
Incline Dumbbell Fly
Cable Crossover
Cable Flys

"Specialty Exercises"
Soto Press
Weighted Push Up

Triceps:

"Checkpoint Lifts"
Close Grip Bench Press
Skullcrusher
Seated Triceps Extension
Standing Triceps Extension

"Assistance Lifts"
Cable Press Down
Cable Rope Press Down
Standing Cable Rope Extension
(overhead)
Reverse Grip Cable Press Down
One Arm Cable Press Down

One Arm Reverse Grip Cable
Press Down
Overhead Dumbbell Extension
1-Arm Overhead Dumbbell
Extension
Incline Dumbell Triceps
Extension

"Specialty Exercises"
Dumbell Pull Overs
Ez Bar Pull Overs
JM Press
Rippetoe Cable Press Down

Back:

"Checkpoint Lifts"
Weighted Chin Up
Weighted Pull Up
Cable Pull Down (Supinated,
Pronated or Neutral Grip)
Powerclean

"Assistance Lifts"
Bent Over Dumbbell Row
1 Arm Dumbbell Row
1 Arm Machine Row
Cable Row
Barbell Row

"Specialty Exercises"
Pedlay Row
Rack Pulls
Barbell Shrugs

Biceps:

"Checkpoint Lifts"
Barbell Curl
EZ bar Curl
Incline Dumbbell Curl
Incline Hammer Curl

"Assistance Lifts"
Cable Curl
Cable Reverse Curl
Ez Bar Reverse Curl
Preacher Curl
Reverse Preacher Curl

"Specialty Exercises"
Zottman Curl
Fat Bar / FatGrip Curl
Fat Bat / FatGrip
Reverse Curl

Legs:

"Checkpoint Lifts"
Squat (any Variation)
Front Squat (Any Variation)
Sumo Deadlift
Weighted Pistol
Bulgarian Split Squat
45 Degree Leg Press

"Assistance Lifts"
Machine Leg Press
Leg Extension
Walking Lunge
Step Up

"Specialty Exercises"
Partial Range Squat
Pause Squat

How To Avoid Injury

Like I mentioned earlier, self-limiting training movements will mitigate a large amount of the risk involved in terms of injury.

These movements, when executed with proper weight progression over adequate amount of time, will keep you below the negative stress threshold.

However, I want to also make sure you eliminate your chance of musculoskeletal injury so you can continue making progress on this protocol well into the future with no problems.

Injury will only come from you trying to progress too quickly, and therefore lifting too much weight before your body is ready to handle it. If your body hasn't adapted properly yet, you put yourself at unnecessary risk by trying to move too quickly through the progression.

Lifting weight that is too heavy will compromise your form, which will expose less-trained muscles and tendons to the training load... areas of your body with less mature neural conditioning, that are not ready to handle the weight.

This is when you get injured.

Remember: this program is all about working with your body, harnessing its natural drive for survival by forcing steady adaptive change. This process requires a lot of patience, but over the course of months and years, you will reap the rewards of a hyper efficient neuromuscular system and superior power and strength. Neuromuscular development takes time, so go into this process with a long-term mindset. Don't rush, and you won't get injured.

You will see that in the same amount of time you spend carefully increasing your weight over this year, that you will be lifting very heavy loads before you know it, while your friends or other regular gym buddies will likely have progressed very little, if at all.

You need to adhere to this patient, methodical increase in exposure to the adaptive stimulus (weight).

Do not make large jumps.

The THOR Program is an advanced lifting program designed to elicit hormonal output. Due to the fact that is designed to be neurally challenging, I recommend all untrained or semi-trained (weekend warrior types) undergo a period of acclimatization before beginning it.

If you are a regular weight lifter with a few years of consistent training under your belt you should be okay beginning the program today.

If you need to undergo this acclimatization phase, however, I highly recommend you do.

Please be honest with yourself on this matter; it hurts only you to try and jump into this too quickly when your body is not ready.

The untrained man will still see steady hormonal gains from the right type of acclimatization training. Studies show that in untrained men, hormonal response is actually higher than in elite athletes for comparable training regimens, until the body is properly acclimatized; so don't worry about not reaping the benefits of THOR immediately. You will still be getting some amazing hormonal outputs. I recommend any of the Beginner and Intermediate training routines from the TestShock Program for this acclimatization period of 1-3 months.

I recommend these workouts because they are still designed to be self-limiting in nature, based around neuromuscular training movements. Your body will get accustomed to this style of training in a way that prepares it for THOR.

This is the best way to eliminate your chance of injury early in your THOR training journey.

Once you begin THOR, I also highly recommend training with a partner or at least making sure you have a spotter available to you on non-machine lifts where you are pushing your boundaries.

For example, let's say on incline bench you are looking to hit a PR of 225 lbs for 5 today. Since this is just a minor increase in the weight you put up last week, and you are well recovered nutritionally and physically, it shouldn't be an issue.

However, you are probably a bit wary of the new milestone psychologically, so I recommend having a spotter available, especially for the final 2 reps, where most people seem to psychologically falter and that final muscle fatigue typically sets in. Just having the spotter is usually enough to help you through the set unassisted, but it is also a nice insurance policy so, if you do falter, you don't drop a 225 lb barbell on your chest.

Why Recovery Is Half The Battle & Should Be Taken As Seriously As Your Training

It is also PARAMOUNT that you take recovery as seriously as you take the actual training.

Most people think training 3 times a week is too little training, and that they need to be in the gym daily lifting to achieve any kind of progress.

This is completely 100% false.

Recall when I mentioned earlier that when you do the wrong type of training, you are either being counterproductive or ineffective. Training more often than necessary, and in doing so neglecting proper recovery, is the definition of counterproductive.

It's no wonder the guys you see (and who recommend) lifting daily are almost always in one of the following two scenarios:

1. Cycling anabolic steroids, pro-hormones, or SARMs

2. Stagnant, lifting the same weight they've been lifting for years, with the essentially the same mediocre physique

To address the steroid issue, guys on steroids can lift more often and recover much faster from their training sessions than guys not using steroids. This is a fact. That have unnaturally high levels of circulating androgens and therefore could do pushups every day as their sole training and still gain muscle. They can also, depending on what they're cycling, workout for hours every day and recover easily.

They're also typically the VAST majority of bloggers, cover models, social media fitness celebrities, and forum posters you see around the fitness online community that recommend and teach people to train every day. They have no problem with it, and they don't know anything different, so it only follows that they would recommend it to others.

However, if you're NOT cycling anabolic steroids, you must not take advice from guys who are.

Your body CANNOT recover as quickly as theirs can.

As a natural lifter, you are biologically limited. You must accept this and use it to your advantage.

You've chosen the path of not completely ruining your endocrine system (good choice) and instead have chosen that you value your hormonal health and long term vitality and you recognize that there are actually some great ways to naturally reach the top-end of testosterone optimization with proper training (ie. THOR), nutrition, and lifestyle techniques.

Recovery is essential to this process.

Nutrition and physical rest & sleep are vital to recovering before hitting your next session.

And trust me, once you are acclimatized and progressing on THOR at full capacity, you will savor the recovery days between training days, not only because the constant progression will always leave you sore, but also because you will become addicted to lifting more weight every week in major movements.

Hitting PRs almost weekly is addicting.

And recovery between training sessions is responsible for 50% of that.

Chapter 6

Cardio

For me, life is continuously being hungry. The meaning of life is not simply to exist, to survive, but to move ahead, to go up, to achieve, to conquer.

— Arnold Schwarzenegger

C ardio is a simple topic. The question of "should I do cardio?" can be answered by an "it depends…" What is your goal?

If your goal is simply to have a good looking physique, then you don't need to do cardio. We've seen this time and again across many different groups of lifters. Resistance training, independent of cardiovascular training, is enough of a stimulus to build a great physique, assuming diet is solid as well.

If your goal is more than just having a great physique, but on top of that physique to also build a healthy, athletic body with some longevity, then I recommend doing specific types of cardio.

The cool thing about cardio is that you can also use specific types of cardio to elicit a hormonal response, as we will soon discuss.

However, some types of cardio are completely counterproductive to your goal of increasing androgen receptor density and binding, and therefore must be avoided.

Any kind of endurance-oriented aerobic cardio should be avoided, to eliminate all risk of chronic cortisol elevation from training. It is far too easy to keep intensity low enough, and duration long enough, with chronic endurance training, to steadily increase circulating cortisol levels over time.

Endurance training is also completely out of line with our goals as THOR adherents, principally. It does absolutely nothing to help you, compromises neural recovery, and therefore must be avoided. Channel that extra energy into lifting heavier weights.

Now that you know what NOT to do, let's talk about what you SHOULD do.

There are a handful of benefits to some specific cardio training:

* Increased ability to utilize oxygen efficiently (which will help you lift heavier over time)

* The rejuvenative effect on cellular turnover & blood circulation (from walking)

* Hormonal response of testosterone and GH to help support an increase in circulating androgen levels

Specific Cardio Recommendation – Walking

Walking is one of the best things you can do for your body. The rejuvenative effects are outstanding to support your recovery and circulation.

I recommend walking 30-60 minutes a day, not just while THOR training but also for the rest of your life.

People generally don't understand that walking should form the base of their fitness.

Walking has been used for literally thousands of years to condition all types of athletes including special operations forces. If it's good enough for them, it's probably good enough for you.

In terms of practical application, walking can be considered the original form of general physical preparedness (GPP). Basically, regardless of the distance or fitness application, walking is the ultimate form of general physical preparedness. It gets your body ready for just about anything, balances the hormones and helps your body resist the many negative effects of a sedentary lifestyle.

Many doctors discuss the problems with being sedentary. An example would be the study cited here that linked each hour per day of TV watching with an additional 18% chance of heart disease and diabetes.

It's really not that you need to move to burn off calories or tone your muscles so much as that the entire endocrine system, digestive system, neuromuscular system etc… has evolved to need a certain amount of movement, particularly walking. Scientists point to the idea that people evolved to get between 3-5 miles a day per walking at a minimum. This is one of the reasons that people have gotten such amazing results with the 10,000 steps per day programs. Basically they puts you at 4.5-5 miles per day of walking which is the high minimum range for the amount of walking humans evolved to perform.

By simply adding a good amount of walking per day you will drastically increase your fitness level if you were far below 10000 steps per day. You will make dieting much easier by avoiding the metabolic derangement you begin to experience at very low activity levels and you will sleep better.

Specific Cardio Recommendation – Sprinting

You'll notice that on the THOR training protocol I advise sprinting.

Sprinting is incredible for facilitating release of testosterone and growth hormone levels.

It's a tired (and completely common sense) argument, so I will only quickly mention it, but just take a look at sprinters, as track athletes.

Their physiques are a testament to the power of the explosive movement to increase circulating androgens which impact muscle density, neural power, and low body fat levels.

Sprinting once a week (I don't recommend sprinting farther than 200m at a time), is an amazing way to keep your body lean, powerful, and athletic in the midst of heavy weight training.

It's also an efficient way to build your lower body and midsection power, especially when weight room movements like heavy back squatting may slow power development.

Sprinting will also facilitate just the right amount of leg hypertrophy, but the limitations of gravity and forward motion will keep your legs from getting bulky. Instead they will be muscular and powerful. You are training for increases in power and explosiveness on THOR, so sprinting is perfect for facilitating this in your lower body muscle groups.

Stand tall when you sprint and hold proper form. You'll get a nice GH flush through the entire body on your sprint days.

Hypoxia

Hypoxia and training under low oxygen density conditions has been the subject of a great deal of research.

This mostly has to do with the adaptations the body makes to low oxygen conditions in relation to exercise performance and endurance.

Since low oxygen conditions are able to induce favorable changes in athlete's physiology, many competitive endurance athletes and coaches have used atmospheric chambers or training at altitude to create the low oxygen conditions needed for these physiological changes to take place.

Out of this research came an interest in hypoxia and its effects on skeletal muscle by diverse groups of competitive and recreational athletes looking to increase strength power and size.

One study that was conducted to measure the effectiveness of hypoxia and strength training had athletes experience low oxygen conditions for periods before and after strength training. What the researchers found was that the strength and size increases were similar between the two groups, but metabolic adaptations were very different.

What changed was the capillary to fiber ratio in the muscles as well as levels of growth hormone in the blood stream measured after training.

Researchers found that the athletes that underwent oxygen deprivation had higher levels of metabolic adaptations in the muscles though they had performed the same exercise. Researchers noted that this could be beneficial in preventing arterial or metabolic related issues such as arterial stiffness.

Basically short term hypoxia is a good way to place acute stress on the circulatory system being worked by your chosen resistance exercise. What's more is that exercise in hypoxic conditions is a proven way to increase growth hormone.

Beyond the ability of hypoxic training to increase growth hormone it has the potential to allow for increased work through the decreased lactic acid levels created under hypoxic conditions.

Hemoglobin is the body's main transporter of both oxygen and carbon dioxide. When either of the two is increased in the blood stream the other one decreases in concentration. In hypoxic conditions carbon dioxide is therefore increased. By simply denying the body oxygen you automatically increase levels of carbon dioxide in the blood stream.

In addition to carbon dioxide's inverse relationship to oxygen, it shares an inverse relationship with lactic acid. As carbon dioxide levels in the blood increase, lactic acid levels fall off. This was first noticed when scientists looked at the blood work and physiological reaction of endurance athletes training at altitude.

Researchers discovered that the lower concentrations of oxygen found at higher altitudes resulted in higher blood levels of carbon dioxide and lower levels of lactic acid.

Unlike endurance exercise which depends heavily on the body's ability to process and transport oxygen, anaerobic exercise depends heavily on the nervous system as well as the body's lactic acid buffering abilities.

Therefore anything that assists the body in clearing lactic acid from the blood stream has the ability to increase the performance of anaerobic muscle tissue.

Further complicating this matter is the idea that endurance athletes are often limited by their body's lactic threshold or anaerobic threshold.

This is the level of muscular action, speed of running, cycling or muscular contraction etc... at which the levels of lactic acid in the blood accumulates fast enough to build up and ultimately limit performance.

If endurance athletes could somehow benefit from higher concentrations of carbon dioxide and its lactic acid lowering effects, they could potentially remove one of the main roadblocks to higher levels of performance. This issue is that high levels of oxygen are required to sustain the intensive aerobic processes taking place during this type of activity.

The situation an endurance athlete performing at their lactate threshold finds himself in is very different from that of an athlete performing resistance training exercise. Think about it, a marathon runner moving at 13 mph will not be able to hold their breath in order to increase the concentration of carbon dioxide and decrease the concentration of lactic acid in the blood. While this could remove one roadblock to higher performance it will create a much larger one in limiting the supply of oxygen to the lungs.

What if we look at this same scenario under conditions which do not rely so heavily on oxygen. Take an extended set of side lateral raises, for example.

During a relatively isolated exercise such as side lateral raises, the contraction of the muscles, even over a relatively long set, will not be limited by the oxygen levels in your blood.

Even a pretty high rep set of an isolation exercise such as a side lateral raise does not cause a large elevation in full body aerobic activity. This allows for a scenario in which hypoxic conditions can be utilized to allow for increased muscular action.

Under normal conditions lactic acid is one of the limiters of muscular actions. One of the ways this works is that lactic acid interferes with the signals the nervous system send to the muscles.

This is one of the reasons why high rep "pump and burn" training is not good for long term muscle growth. The lactic acid produced by this type of training inhibits the nervous system and does little to enhance the changes that can cause long term muscle growth.

For the most part this type of high rep training is good for causing acute metabolic changes to the muscle and some sarcoplasmic hypertrophy.

However, if we use this type of training under hypoxic conditions it can be used as a novel stimulus to increase growth hormone levels or potentially allow for increased work – which is extremely important for hormonal adaptive release.

The ability of hypoxic training to increase the amount of work a muscle can perform is the result I am truly interested in and the reason that I have been experimenting with this type of training in my own workouts.

The best way to apply this type of hypoxic training is to the end of your workout as a bonus or burnout set for specific isolated muscles.

The reason I like to do this is twofold. First training heavy all the time is taxing. Outside of a few benchmark exercises which you should use to gauge progress, you need to the movements you are doing.

What's more is that on exercises such as side lateral raises that depend on discrete increases in weight of up to 5 lbs per dumbbell, progression via weight used is the least desirable model.

Exercises such as these that do not lend themselves to huge jumps in weight are just the type that can benefit from hypoxic training.

The easiest way to benefit from this type of training is to simply do a "breath-hold" set. The idea is to breath in through your nose perform one extended set, usually 8-12 reps, and then slowly exhale through the mouth slowly.

You can wait until the end of the set to exhale or slowly exhale as you get toward completion depending on your fitness levels and levels of familiarity with the technique.

Alternatively you can hold your breath as long as possible before the beginning of a set and begin as soon as you start. You will need to experiment with both techniques to see what you are able to do most effectively.

Millet G, Bentley DJ, Roels B, Mc Naughton LR, Mercier J, Cameron-Smith D. "Effects of intermittent training on anaerobic performance and MCT transporters in athletes," *PLoS One*. 2014 May 5;9(5):e95092. doi: 10.1371/ journal.pone.0095092. ECollection 2014.

Robach P1, Bonne T, Flück D, Bürgi S, Toigo M, Jacobs RA, Lundby C. "Hypoxic Training: Effect on Mitochondrial Function and Aerobic Performance in Hypoxia," *Med Sci Sports Exerc*. 2014 Mar 26.

Chapter 7

The Training Protocols

Life's a garden, dig it.

— Joe Dirt

Explosive control is the name of the game here.

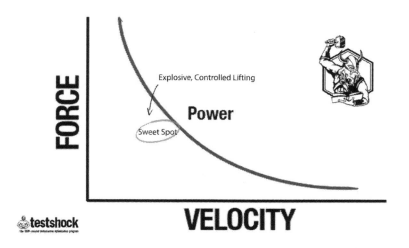

You want to control the *release* (ie. the opposing motion of the lift itself) of the lift just enough to hold great form and stabilize your lift, however you do not want to control it so much that it is itself giving you resistance – if that makes sense.

The following breakdown is the THOR weekly program, as it currently stands.

This protocol will allow you to make consistent increases in major lifts week after week, going into your week 4 of the cycle – the consolidation week, where you will drop the volume but consolidate your progress with heavy lift variations.

It'll all make sense in a minute.

Macro Progression-Consolidation Cycle

- **Week 1:** +

- **Week 2:** ++

- **Week 3:** +++

- **Week 4:** Consolidation

Rinse and repeat. Over each cycle you will be stronger and stronger. You are creating a "new normal" like I discussed earlier, through steady forced adaptation to continually heavier weight through movement, and lifting in a way to facilitate power generation will allow you to hit the sweet spot when it comes to hormonal response elicited from the stimulus.

The following are the weekly protocols.

5 Day Split

On the 5 day split, for those of you who enjoy going to the gym during the weekdays, I recommend doing less volume during your workout sessions so you can facilitate full neural recovery from one session to the next, as proper recovery is so paramount to your success and the sustainability of your progress.

For example, within our guidelines, you would opt for 2-4 sets of one checkpoint lift at 5-8 reps, 2-4 sets of between 2-4 assistance lifts at 6-12 reps, and 0-1 specialty lifts.

Do not make your decision of how many assistance lifts to perform based on any rigid rules, but rather listen your the current state of your body at the time of training. If you're feeling tired or low energy, we recommend doing less volume. If you're feeling great, do more.

Listening to the natural ebb and flow of your body will, over time, help you sustain progress without burnout.

Take ample recovery time between sets. It is of our opinion that if you can jump straight back into another set without much rest, then you aren't lifting enough (ie. doing enough work) on your sets, and should increase the load.

Break your 5 day split into the following break down.

Day 1: Chest & Tricep & Trap focus

Day 2: Back and Bicep focus

Day 3: Full Body and Leg focus

Day 4: Shoulder & Trap Focus

Day 5: Sprinting and Calisthenic focus

Now let's look at some examples of those days. I will fill in the Training Log with these example workout sessions so you can visualize everything in the right framework.

Note: Remember to perform your lifts with a controlled explosive motion. Using weighted dips for an example, use control going down, and explode up.

Day 1: Chest Focus

FOCUS: Chest/Tri/Traps	SET 1	SET 2	SET 3
Date: 00/00/00			
CHECKPOINT LIFT(S)			
Weighted Dips	5 x 150	6 x 135	8 x 100
ASSISTANCE LIFT(S)			
Flat DB Fly	8 x 45	8 x 45	8 x 45
Cable Pressdown	8 x 110	8 x 110	8 x 110
Seated Machine Fly	8 x 190	8 x 190	8 x 190
DB Shrugs	12 x 120s	12 x 120s	12 x 120s
SPECIALTY LIFT			
Explosive Pushups	8	8	8
NOTES:			

Day 2: Back & Bicep Focus

FOCUS: Back/Biceps	SET 1	SET 2	SET 3
Date: 00/00/00			
CHECKPOINT LIFT(S)			
Weighted Chin-ups	5 x 150	6 x 135	8 x 100
ASSISTANCE LIFT(S)			
Cable Row	8 x 150	8 x 150	8 x 150
Machine Curls	8 x 110	8 x 110	8 x 110
1 Arm DB Row	8 x 90	8 x 90	8 x 90
SPECIALTY LIFT			
NOTES:			
Feeling a bit tired today			
Kept volume lower			

Day 3: Full Body & Leg Focus

FOCUS: Full body/Legs	SET 1	SET 2	SET 3
Date: 00/00/00			
CHECKPOINT LIFT(S)			
Sumo Deadlift	5 x 300	6 x 270	8 x 240
ASSISTANCE LIFT(S)			
Weighted pistol	6 x 45	8 x 45	8 x 45
Glute press	8 x 110	8 x 110	8 x 110
Walking Lunge w/DBs	8 x 60DBs	8 x 60DBs	8 x 60DBs
SPECIALTY LIFT			
Box Jumps		10	10
NOTES:			

Day 4: Shoulder & Trap Focus

FOCUS: Shoulder/Traps	SET 1	SET 2	SET 3	SET 4
Date: 00/00/00				
CHECKPOINT LIFT(S)				
Standing BB Overhead Press	5 x 170	6 x 150	8 x 135	
ASSISTANCE LIFT(S)				
Bent arm lateral cable raise	12 x 20	12 x 20	12 x 20	12 x 20
Barbell behind the neck raise	8 x 110	8 x 110	8 x 110	
DB Shrugs	12 x 120s	12 x 120s	12 x 120s	
SPECIALTY LIFT				
NOTES:				

Page 98

Day 5: Sprinting & Calisthenic Focus

A	B	C	D
FOCUS: Sprinting/calisthenics	**SET 1**	**SET 2**	**SET 3**
Date: 00/00/00			
CHECKPOINT LIFT(S)			
Track sprints	5x100 meters		
Jump knee tucks	2x10		
ASSISTANCE LIFT(S)			
Muscle ups	12	10	8
Clap pull ups	8	8	8
Clap push ups	8	8	8
SPECIALTY LIFT			
NOTES:			

3 Day Split

On the 3 day split, for those of you who can't hit the gym daily - maybe you work long hours and don't want to structure your life around training, I recommend doing more volume during your workout sessions so you can really push your body into an adaptive state on the two big weight training days and the one heavier volume sprint/calisthenics day.

Since you're not training daily you MUST push yourself hard.

Many guys fall into this false line of thinking that "more" is better in terms of how often you train. This is a lie. Doing "more" isn't better, lifting more is.

If you train with so much volume and frequency that your lifts are mediocre because you never fully recover from the previous session, then you aren't ever really forcing your body to adapt to anything - it's just going through the motions. There's no reason for it to release hormonal surges to adapt to the training. Typically, guys in this situation will actually find long term chronic cortisol elevation - which is directly opposite of what you want.

Many guys think 2-3 days of training per week wouldn't be effective for making gains. They're wrong. If you're not making gains, you're not lifting enough weight.

A friend of mine has been doing THOR since it was released in February 2016. He only hits the weight room 2x a week, since he works a full time job as the CEO of a startup and also is a single father of two.

When he trains though, he pushes himself hard, and is fully present. In just a few months of 2x a week lifting he has progressed from using 70lb - 120lb DBs on incline bench, and from 195 to 250 x 5 on his incline barbell bench press, for example. On just two days a week. He's also lost 20lbs of body fat and visibly gained considerable muscle.

The lower-frequency works well for him considering how busy the rest of his life is, but when he trains, he focuses on progression, and now he's lifting more than most guys will ever lift.

So if you're hitting the gym less frequently, you <u>must</u> lift heavy. Stop being dainty and go for the "full stack" mentality.

For example, within our guidelines, you would opt for 3-4 sets of <u>two</u> checkpoint lifts at 5-8 reps, 3-4 sets of between <u>4</u> assistance lifts at 6-12 reps, and 1 specialty lifts.

<u>Break your 3 day split into the following break down.</u>

Workout A: Chest, Shoulder, Tricep & Trap focus

Workout B: Back and Bicep, Trap and Leg focus

Workout C: Sprinting and Calisthenic focus

Now let's look at some examples of those days. I will fill in the Training Log with these example workout sessions so you can visualize everything in the right framework.

Note: Remember to perform your lifts with a controlled explosive motion. Using weighted dips for an example, use control going down, and explode up.

Give yourself at least one day of full rest between each of these sessions.

Workout A: Chest, Shoulder, Tricep & Trap focus:

A	B	C	D
FOCUS: Workout A	**SET 1**	**SET 2**	**SET 3**
Date: 00/00/00			
CHECKPOINT LIFT(S)			
Incline DB Bench press	5 x 120s	6 x 110s	8 x 90s
Standing BB Overhead press	5 x 170	6 x 150	8 x 135
ASSISTANCE LIFT(S)			
Flat DB Flys	8 x 45s	8 x 45s	8 x 45s
Bent arm lateral raise with DBs	8 x 50s	8 x 50s	8 x 50s
Cable pressdown	10 x full stack	10 x full stack	10 x full stack
DB Shrugs	12 x 120s	12 x 120s	12 x 120s
SPECIALTY LIFT			
Clap Push Ups	5 x 10		
NOTES:			
cooldown stretching, foam rollers			
back bridging	5 x 30 seconds		

Workout B: Back and Bicep, Trap and Leg focus

FOCUS: Workout B	SET 1	SET 2	SET 3
Date: 00/00/00			
CHECKPOINT LIFT(S)			
Weighted Chin-ups	5 x 135	6 x 110	8 x 90
Sumo deadlift	5 x 350	6 x 315	8 x 285
ASSISTANCE LIFT(S)			
Cable row	8 x 150	8 x 150	8 x 150
Glute Press back machine	8 x full stack	8 x full stack	8 x full stack
Machine curls	10 x 180	8 x 180	8 x 180
DB Shrugs	12 x 120s	12 x 120s	12 x 120s
SPECIALTY LIFT			
Calf raises	8 x 150	8 x 150	8 x 150
NOTES:			
cooldown stretching, foam rollers			
back bridging	5 x 30 seconds		

Workout C: Sprinting & Calisthenics focus

A	B	C	D	
FOCUS: Workout C	**SET 1**	**SET 2**	**SET 3**	
Date: 00/00/00				
CHECKPOINT LIFT(S)				
Track sprints	10x100 meters			
Jump knee tucks	2x10			
ASSISTANCE LIFT(S)				
Muscle ups		12	10	8
Clap pull ups		8	8	8
Clap push ups		8	8	8
Burpees	5x10			
SPECIALTY LIFT				
NOTES:				

So there you have it. Those are some good sample training weeks to help get you on the road to success with THOR.

You can use those, or create your own according to the guidelines.

Our recommendation is that you spend 1 month (consolidation cycle) at a time doing the same weekly routine.

Every month you can switch things up slightly with the Checkpoint and Assistance lifts when you feel like your progress may be stalling on something. This will help emphasize the right movements and muscle groups, while still progressing forward without plateaus.

Chapter 8

A Novel Nutrition Plan

You miss 100% of the shots you don't take.

— Wayne Gretzky

With the THOR program we advise you to focus on consuming balanced nutrition. By balanced nutrition I am talking about making sure you get enough of all three macronutrients.

If you are used to low carbohydrate dieting or low fat dieting you are going to have to change your mindset. Most of the diets that focus on restricting any one macronutrient are based on short term results.

Often these results are some specific effect on the body, or even just making the dieter feel like their diet is effective.

As I mentioned at the start of the program I am looking at your body as a system. Diet being one part of that system it should be in support and service of all the other parts of that system. This is where the radical idea of balancing macronutrients comes into play.

Diets that restrict any macronutrient are not appropriate for testosterone enhancement. It has been shown time and time again that restricting carbohydrates and fats in particular will inhibit your body's production of testosterone.

What is even more astounding is the negative effect high protein diets can have on testosterone levels. If you were to follow most of the mainstream physique building advice you would be setting yourself up for hormonal issues, low testosterone in particular.

Of course this is not a concern for many of the fitness celebrities who get their testosterone from external sources. Since we are concerned with absolutely maximizing natural testosterone production you need a diet that facilitates maximum hormonal output.

Any short term benefit you may have gotten from a specific cutting or bulking protocol will be far outpaced by having consistently high levels of the body's most potent anabolic hormones.

In study after study, moderate to high carbohydrate diets outperform low carbohydrate productions in maintaining and increasing testosterone levels. In low carbohydrate dieters, as carbohydrates are increased levels of GnRH, the hormone that begins the cascade of events that leads to testosterone production is increased.

When athletes are put on high and low carbohydrate diets, those on the higher carbohydrate diets have consistently lower levels of cortisol over time. Finally, multiple studies have shown consistently higher free testosterone levels in moderate carbohydrate dieters over time.

Similarly low fat diets have been shown to inhibit testosterone production. When looking at fats you need to consider the three main types of fats that people consume, monounsaturated, polyunsaturated and saturated fats.

In terms of enhancing testosterone production you want to keep the ratio of monounsaturated and saturated to polyunsaturated fatty acids as high as possible.

This is because polyunsaturated fatty acids do not increase testosterone as much as the other two types of fats. Many studies have even shown that they have an inhibitory effect on testosterone.

I will get into specific recommendations for fat containing foods, but for starters eggs, avocados, steak, coconut oil and olive oil are some good basic sources of monounsaturated and saturated fat.

Finally protein which is both the most important and least important macronutrient needs to be considered. Protein is the most important because it is a complex macronutrient that is vitally important component of cell growth.

It is also the least important because the body does not need a great deal of protein on a day to day basis. Speaking generally, protein is most useful as a building block for the body's various cells and tissues.

Unlike fats and carbohydrates which are easily used for energy, protein requires a great deal of processing to be broken down and used as energy by the body.

In fact, when the body tries to use protein for energy in place of fats or carbohydrates it expends a large percentage of the potential energy it can get from each protein molecule just breaking it down.

Protein Molecules...Hard to Break Down

Using an analogy, let's say you are camping and you have a campfire that you usually keep going with charcoal and wood.

Everything is going fine and your campfire is burning bright. One day you get tired of having to constantly use wood and charcoal.

You get the idea to use your tent to keep the fire going instead. You walk over to the tent, snap the polls out and toss the whole thing in the fire.

You notice that it doesn't burn as well as the wood or the charcoal and ends up kinda making a mess putting off a bunch of black smoke etc... This is kind of like what happens when you force the body to use protein as one of its main sources of energy.

It is forced to break down the complex protein molecules for energy. Not only is this wasteful but it creates a bunch of nasty byproducts.

Your body prefers getting energy from carbs and fats.

When the body easily find enough energy from fats and carbohydrates and uses most of the protein it gets for building other types of tissue.

It also reduces the stress the body is under as it does not have to break down complex protein molecules for all of its energy needs.

Research into diet composition shows that high protein diets reliably reduce testosterone levels.

If that wasn't bad enough chronically over consuming protein in place of carbohydrates in particular can lead to an altered testosterone to cortisol ratio making it harder to lose fat and gain muscle.

It might seems obvious to most people, but you have to lower protein intake in order to make room in your diet for fats and carbohydrates.

This is because you cannot simply eat more off all three macronutrients.

This would cause you to be consistently over your caloric requirements which would cause weight gain, reduced insulin sensitivity and a number of other problems. Your takeaway from this section should be that your diet should be balanced.

I recommend starting with around 20% of calories coming from protein, 40% coming from fats and 40% coming from carbohydrates.

Keep in mind that this is just a starting point and you will have to play around from there to figure out what works best for you.

Priming The Anabolic Environment Through Fasting

Fasting has been shown to directly influence hormone secretion in men.

In large part your nutritional status and the quality of your sleep will determine the amount of growth hormone that is released in your body.

Basically when insulin levels are lower in your body, growth hormone levels become higher. This is one of the biggest reasons that some people seem to magically burn fat once they cut out foods that greatly increase circulating insulin levels.

One of the reasons that fasting is so effective at increasing growth hormone is that fasting requires you to completely forgo any intake of calories.

This means that any healthy individual will see a decrease in circulating insulin and an increase in circulating growth hormone.

The confusion many people experience with other types of diets is that they are led to believe that certain foods are alright to eat and that they will not increase insulin levels. Even many diet gurus believe that certain foods, especially low carbohydrate foods will not increase insulin levels.

What this fails to take into account is the insulin index. Basically this is a measure of how much insulin is released in response to the intake of certain foods.

Traditionally researchers looked at the amount of carbohydrate in certain foods or the glycemic load of certain foods to determine how much insulin they would release.

This represents a best guess as it correlates carbohydrates with insulin directly. The insulin index instead measures the actual levels of insulin released in the body in response to certain foods.

What researchers found was enlightening.

For example, it was found that beef, a traditionally low carbohydrate food with a low glycemic index raised insulin levels more than many high glycemic index foods. While there are many ways to interpret this data, the point is that many types of foods raise insulin levels regardless of carbohydrate content.

This is another reason the THOR Program focuses on calories overall and not specific macronutrients or the glycemic index of foods.

Trying to manipulate individual variables in a complex system results in lackluster results. Instead you should focus on a few huge levers like overall calorie intake.

This is most easily accomplished through the short daily fast.

GH, Testosterone and Hormonal Synergy

The point of saying all this is to reinforce the idea that focusing on overall calories, and periods of complete abstinence from calories are one of the only surefire ways to get a consistently strong output of growth hormone in the body (along with adequate REM sleep and proper training).

You want to be regularly experiencing these releases of growth hormone in order to enhance testosterone production and maintain a low level of body fat.

Growth hormone does this by working synergistically with testosterone to enhance body composition. This happens because the two hormones are both supportive of one and other.

When testosterone levels are increased growth hormone levels are directly affected and are increased.

When growth hormone is increased, testosterone in indirectly increased.

This happens when growth hormone increases gonadotropins which cause the testes to increase their production of sperm and testosterone.

Growth hormone's effects on testosterone are so profound that both testosterone's androgenic and anabolic properties are inhibited when growth hormone levels are below normal.

The point is that anything that increases growth hormone is going to have a positive impact on testosterone and its enhancement of primary and secondary sex characteristics.

Short daily fasts are a nearly guaranteed way to experience elevated growth hormones levels without the more drastic spikes in cortisol that are seen in prolonged fasting or starvation diets.

Secondary Benefits of Fasting

Fasting has also been proven to induce autophagy in the body. This is the body's internal process of cellular turnover.

The body basically has the ability to use some of its older more damaged cells for energy and raw materials. The body is able to break down cells that it no longer needs to use for other processes.

What's interesting about this process is that the body selectively targets cells that have excessive damage from things like free radicals.

Therefore the body is left with a higher percentage of relatively new cells every time you experience increased level of autophagy.

Many diet gurus have attempted to increase levels of autophagy in the body by including special low protein days in their diets.

Instead of messing around with high and low calorie days, high and low carbohydrate days and high and low protein days I suggest a simple daily fast.

This process initiates a daily cycle of autophagy, increased growth hormone output as well as a steady decrease in insulin. Instead of messing around with spiking different macronutrients on different days you simply experience all of the benefits at once with simple daily fasts.

While you may be able to maximize cellular turnover, insulin levels or growth hormone levels ever so slightly with a more complex process, having something you can do every day will benefit you more in the long run.

Simply including daily fasting into your routine gets you 80-90% of the benefits of any more complicated dietary strategy. Since you will be able to do it every day it will net you far more benefits than any on again off again strategy the diet gurus are claiming.

While you may be scratching your head as "not eating" seems like too simple a strategy to work, keep in mind that it is one component of a lifestyle you are building to take advantage of every testosterone enhancing habit you can have.

While intermittent fasting is not appropriate in all circumstances, the recommendations made in THOR are for the average member of the TestShock audience.

This means you are probably a guy that is not performing hard physical labor during the day. You should be performing some low volume strength training and doing some low intensity cardio and mobility to maintain your functionality.

For this type of guy, short daily intermittent fasting is perfect.

Recommended THOR Diet Protocol

Okay now you're probably wondering what you should do every day when it comes to eating & fasting.

I will break it all down in this section right now.

And once again, I'm going to make this very simple. So simple, in fact, that many guys will likely feel genuine "fear" – why? Because everyone is so used to complicated "guru" nonsense when it comes to dietary recommendations that we've begun finding comfort in the complications... we're so used to complicated nonsense that we fear something simple.

"There's no way something simple could work for me," we think. "I'm special."

Like I said in the beginning of this chapter, I promote balanced nutrition.

For some reason, nowadays, promoting balance is heretical, or radical – which seems insane to me, but hey, at least you're not going to follow all that nonsensical "fad" dieting anymore if you believe me.

If you're tired of yo-yo'ing, lackluster results in the gym, and a soft physique, then I implore you to please give this simple plan a shot.

You will – guaranteed – find it refreshing.

And liberating.

Freedom is important.

Here's what to do:

1. Fast daily, and eat 2 meals within a 6-8 hour window. You can be flexible on this eating window, since many people have varying schedules.

2. The 2 meals are:

   a) The Macronutrient Meal (ie. Strong Meal)

       i. This meal is focused on getting the proper macronutrients into your system. You are fueling your training and recovery with this meal, specifically (that's an easy way to think about this).

       ii. Eat 1-2lbs of quality meat.

       iii. Remainder of meal is carbs and fat.

       iv. This meal is great for flexibility, especially when fasting all day. Many guys can consume up to 2000 calories here or more, depending on body size (for example, I am 210 lbs so I can eat a massive meal here). Eat like a f-cking Viking King. I've become a fan of ordering two entrees at restaurants...

       v. **The Strong Meal** keeps you non-rigid. Go out for burgers and fries, steaks and potatoes, burritos, etc. Don't eat shit food, eat quality food. But you don't have to be rigid. You can live like a normal social person, and you can eat like a man – not a bird. Life and good food are meant to be enjoyed!

       vi. If you focus on eating 80% high quality macro sources in this meal (ie. monounsaturated fats, starches, organic free range meats), you not only have a little wiggle room for other things like alcohol or an occasional dessert, but you also keep peace of mind and the flexibility necessary for actually maintaining progress over time. If you have problems with binge eating, you will quickly see how simple it is to overcome when you add the flexibility.

b) The Micronutrient Meal

vii. The sole purpose of this meal is to provide your body with all of the micronutrients it needs (on top of the Macro Meal) in order to properly produce the hormones you are working so hard to optimize.

viii. This meal is also very simple.

ix. I recommend smoothies as an easy way to get all of the nutrition into an easy-to-consume format.

x. For example, I recently had my micronutrient analysis from **ResetYourself.com/testshock** and found out my key vitamin and mineral deficiencies that I need to eliminate. This meal is my opportunity every day to work toward getting rid of these deficiencies, then keeping my body topped off with amazing nutrients. My favorite Micro Meal right now is a smoothie with 2 bananas (for potassium & to eliminate cramping in my legs), a good organic greens powder, a full avocado, 2 brazil nuts, fish oil with Vitamin D3, and Gerolsteiner mineral water (high mineral content in magnesium, potassium, calcium and sodium). I call this Micronutrient Meal my "affordable health insurance policy."

3. To many guys, this plan is music to their ears. To others, they're freaking out right now. Probably for one of the following two reasons:

a) *"I can't eat that much in the Strong Meal."*

    i.   Please stop complaining about eating. Most men (and women) can easily eat 1500 – 2000 calories – or more – down with no problem. Consider this: your lack of progress in muscle gain and in your lifts over your life is almost certainly entirely due to your lack of devotion to getting proper nutritional "fuel" to accommodate those gains. You have a choice now whether you want to continue in the same old patterns, or to choose to be better than that. Remember: "force adaptive change." If you must, feel free to break this into more than one meal. The important thing is the fasting window. But the fewer collective insulin spikes, the better for your GH and T over time.

b) *"Don't I need to eat more protein to protect my gains??"*

    i.   You don't need more than 1-2 lbs of quality meat per day. There will be days when you crave more meat, and days when you crave less. Listen to your appetite. Your body is intelligent. It knows what it needs. If you really don't believe me, then go ahead and drink some BCAAs to ease your mind. Optimizing your T, GH, and DHT levels will do FAR MORE for your gains than some arbitrary protein number you feel you need to adhere to because a protein powder company website installed some fear in you that you'll go "catabolic" if you don't eat more and more of their protein. ***You know what's catabolic... low testosterone.***

4. No – you do not need to count calories or macros if you don't want to.

a) There is definitely value in counting macros and calories if you're new to the fitness journey. You must know what you're working with in terms of quantities so you don't overeat or undereat. Energy in vs. out is a very real thing – I'm not saying calories don't matter. I'm saying, psychologically, you don't need to count them every meal if you're experienced enough to intuit overall food intake.

b) Most people reading this right now are likely experienced in fitness and lifting. You are fully capable of eyeballing foods and generally knowing how many calories or macros you're consuming. If you find comfort in counting, by all means please continue.

c) However, if you are like me, and you find constant counting to be incessantly draining and annoying and you want to live a flexible existence, then you don't have to count – as long as you can "eyeball" your food and remain committed to one thing: DON'T OVEREAT.

d) You can still have amazing progress with this protocol if you're training hard every session and eating according to the simple guidelines I've outlined above – without counting calories or macros.

5. In terms of supplements, see the supplement chapter.

6. I personally recommend and prefer using a quality Pre-Workout drink on this type of fasting protocol, before my training.

a) Criteria for a good pre-workout drink is to include Creatine, Caffeine, Betaine (Estrogen Methylator), and Amino Acids. I also have become enamored with Beta-Hydroxybutarate (BHB) pre training due to the mountain of research showing how effective it is at increasing oxygen efficiency in training.

Also, adaptogens are great to take before training. Again, see the supplements chapter for more information.

7. To help you out with shopping, you can find a 30 testosterone foods grocery list on AnabolicMen.com.

"

If you're tired of yo-yo'ing, lackluster results in the gym, and a soft physique, then I implore you to please give this simple plan a shot.

Chapter 9

Intelligent Supplementation

Plans are only good intentions unless they degenerate into hard work.

— Peter Drucker

We've become quite fond of a handful of supplements that have real research behind their claims. We use these in our own lives and have felt amazing since starting most of them, especially things like Boron, ashwagandha, and phosphatidylserine.

While there are a number of different supplements we have recommended in the past, we are going to narrow down the selection a bit for this program.

One of the complaints we have gotten from clients and in the forum is that guys are not sure where to start supplement wise.

Over the course of the last couple of years we have highlighted a number of our favorite vitamin and mineral formulas as well as the most potent testosterone boosting supplements.

Guys want simple solutions to the problem of what supplements to take.

As many of you know we have been working on a number of supplements we know can outperform anything that is on the market in terms of altering testosterone to cortisol balance in your favor.

If you have been following our work you should know that testosterone to cortisol balance is one of the keys to maintaining a large amount of muscle mass and keeping body fat levels low.

Therefore we have focused my supplementation efforts around positively impacting this ratio.

We will talk a little bit about what makes <u>Testro-X</u> our testosterone enhancing supplement the best on the market. We also have an "Androgen Receptor Optimization Stack" for sale on the Anabolic Men Marketplace right now that includes everything you need to really optimize the results of your THOR training, supplementation-wise.

http://store.anabolicmen.com

Testro–X

During these years of running the Anabolic Men website, several supplement manufacturers have asked us to:

- *Formulate a supplement for them.*
- *Promote their supplements on our site.*
- *And even bash their competitors on our articles.*

However, we have never done any of the things above. Simply because we have never found a supplement which we could fully trust and promote as the #1 testosterone booster. And obviously, were not in the business of smearing other companies reputation for our own (or someones else's) gain.

But now as the AM website has stabilized its place as the leading men's hormonal health resource, we are finally able to actually formulate our own supplements…

…With complete control of the quality of the ingredients, the use of the ingredients, and the dosaging of the ingredients.

This allowed us to finally produce the #1 natural testosterone booster supplement on the market. And if you look through the ingredients and the research behind them below, I think you'll agree with us:

The Perfect Formulation

You can see the ingredient label of Testro-X:

Supplement Facts		
Serving Size: 3 Capsules		
Servings Per Container: 30		
Amount Per Serving		%Daily Value
Magnesium (as Magnesium Citrate)	150 mg	38 %
Zinc (as Zinc Gluconate)	15 mg	100 %
KSM-66® Organic Ashwagandha Root Extract	400 mg	*
Forskohlii Root Extract	250 mg	*
Inositol	200 mg	*
Glycine	200 mg	*
L-Theanine	100 mg	*
Boron (as Boron Citrate)	10 mg	*
Bioperine® Black Pepper Fruit Extract	10 mg	*
* Daily Value not established		

…Unlike many brands manufacturing supplements for increasing testosterone levels, we don't hide behind proprietary blends.

Our ingredients and where they are derived are easily accessible information. We also refuse to use ingredients that aren't proven in science or inhibit some other crucial hormones or enzymes in the body (like 5-ar or DHT).

This is why we decided NOT TO include the following common ingredients:

- *Tribulus terrestris (it doesn't work)*
- *Maca root (it doesn't work either)*
- *Fenugreek (it only raises T because it inhibits DHT)*
- *Saw palmetto (same story as with fenugreek)*
- *D-Aspartic acid (which actually lowers testosterone).*

Here's what we DID include:

Magnesium Citrate

Magnesium can benefit testosterone levels by reducing the levels of sex hormone binding globulin (SHBG).

When SHBG is inhibited, more free-testosterone remains bioactive in the bloodstream and is able to bind into receptor sites.

This is likely the reason why magnesium supplementation and high magnesium levels in the serum are consistently linked to:

- *Higher free-testosterone levels in test-tube studies.*
- *Higher free-testosterone levels in exercising men.*
- *Higher testosterone levels in elderly males.*
- *Positively correlated with anabolic hormones in review studies.*
- *And deficiency – as to be expected – is linked to lowered testosterone.*

Magnesium is highly beneficial for male hormonal health, which is why we decided to include 150mg of well absorbing magnesium citrate into the formula of Testro-X (no higher amount since mega-dosing magnesium is associated with gastric upset, and 150mg on top of average diet is well enough for benefits).

Zinc Gluconate

Zinc is without a doubt the most important mineral for healthy testosterone production.

Aside from being one of the 24 essential micronutrients for human survival and regulating more than 100 bodily enzymes, zinc plays a crucial role in the producion of testosterone, in its utilization by the androgen receptor sites, in DHT production, and at keeping estrogen levels low.

Here's some research about the importance of zinc for hormonal optimization:

- *Supplementation results in higher total and free testosterone and thyroid hormones in exercising men.*
- *Supplementation results in higher total T, free T, and thyroid hormones T3 and T4 in sedentary subjects.*
- *Correcting zinc deficiency has been found to lead to rapid and significant increases in testosterone and DHT levels.*
- *Animal studies have found zinc supplementation to elevate LH levels, testosterone levels, and thyroid hormones.*
- *One study noted that zinc deficiency led to 59% reduction in androgen receptors (36% of those being in testicles).*

There are three extremely bio-available forms of zinc to use in supplementation: picolinate, citrate, and gluconate. We decided to go with 15mg dose of zinc gluconate for Testro-X, as it's known to be the form of zinc containing the lowest amounts of cadmium (a testosterone lowering heavy-metal found in high amounts on low quality zinc supplements).

KSM-66 Ashwagandha

Ashwagandha (Withania Somnifera) is primarily used in the Indian herbal medicine.

Therefore one could think that its effects are not proven in science and only folklores told by the neighborhood shaman…

…But fear not, there actually is Western medicine clinical research behind this herb.

Just take a look at these;

- *Several studies have found ashwagandha to reduce feelings of stress, as well as significantly lower the levels of the stress hormone cortisol.*
- *Ashwagandha has been associated with significant increases in sperm quality and testosterone levels on infertile subjects (up to 40% in 90 days).*
- *In a non-sponsored peer-reviewed study with 57 young healthy male subjects, ashwagandha supplementation raised the average testosterone levels from 630 ng/dL to 726 ng/dL.*

The highest-quality ashwagandha on the market is a patented water-extract called KSM-66 Ashwagandha, we decided to include a potent 400mg dose of it in Testro-X based on the dosages used in majority of the human studies.

Forskohlii Root Extract

Forskohlii root extract (Forskolin), rose to popularity after the notorious fool Dr. Oz proclaimed that it would be a "magical fat-loss miracle".

This obviously was just hype to sell the product, and even though Forskolin works by stimulating certain enzymes necessary for fat oxidization, it isn't exactly as effective as Oz claims.

Now, although that sneaky salesman of a doctor has done his best to make forskolin look like a scam, there actually is some scientifically sound benefits for the root in terms of testosterone optimization.

For instance:

- *Forskolin is well known for increasing the levels of intracellular cAMP (cyclic adenosine monophosphate).*
- *Increased cAMP is known for its stimulatory effect on testosterone production and androgen receptor (AR) activation.*
- *Forskolin in cell-culture studies has been linked to significant and consistent increases in testosterone.*
- *250mg's of Forskolin was able to increase T levels by 33% when compared to placebo in overweight males.*

Based on the human study which showed nice increases in testosterone levels, we decided to include 250mg's of high-quality Forskolin in Testro-X formulation.

Boron Citrate

You may or may not have heard about boron before.
It's a trace-mineral, not considered absolutely essential for survival, and honestly, not that popular as a supplement.

Here at Anabolic Men we absolutely love boron, and we believe it deserves more attention than what it is getting now…

…Here's why:

- *In rodent studies, boron has been found to dose-dependently increase testosterone levels.*
- *6mg's of boron for 2 months in human subjects was associated with a nice 29% increase in testosterone levels.*
- *10mg's of boron for 7 days in humans was able to increase free-testosterone by 28%, while reducing estrogen by 39% and boosting DHT by 10%.*

Boron deserves more attention as an essential trace-mineral for maintaining male hormonal balance. We are proud to include 10mg's of highest-quality boron citrate in Testro-X.

Luteinizing Hormone Surge Blend

When your body naturally produces testosterone, the whole cascade starts from the brain substrate called hypothalamus, which releases a hormone called GnRH...

...GnRH then stimulates the release of luteinizing hormone (LH) from the pituitary gland...

...Which then travels down to your testicles via the spine and triggers the leydig cells to synthesize testosterone.

Our idea with the specific *"LH Surge Blend"*, was to identify natural compounds that can stimulate the release of GnRH and LH, for higher amount of natural testosterone production.

- *That's why we included 200mg's of inositol, a precursor needed for the natural synthesis of GnRH.*
- *That's also why we included 100mg's of L-theanine, which excites the GABA-neurons in the brain and stimulates GnRH release.*
- *And finally the blend was completed with 200mg's of glycine, which increases the pulsatile release of GnRH.*

Bioperine®

Bioperine is a patented extract of the black pepper fruit. Although there's animal research suggesting that black pepper fruit extract may be beneficial for androgenic hormones in rodents, we didn't include bioperine in Testro-X because of those studies. Instead, we formulated bioperine into the supplement as it is known to significantly enhance the absorption of many herbs, minerals, vitamins, and amino-acids.

We wanted to make sure that the ingredients in the supplement, actually absorb into the body to provide real effects.

Hence the bioperine, and if it boosts testosterone as it did in the rat studies, that's obviously just another plus.

When we say that Testro-X is the best testosterone booster on the market, we're not joking around.

Every ingredient in this supplement has been scientifically proven to either increase testosterone levels or improve the absorption of other ingredients.

No shady herbs with baseless claims, no hiding behind propietary blends and ineffective dosages...

...Just 100% research-backed men's health supplements.

Testro-X is now available for sale on our Marketplace at
store.anabolicmen.com

Choline Bitartrate

A key nutrient for the human diet is choline. Choline, commonly grouped in the B vitamin family, is integral to many human body functions some of which are brain, liver, cellular, and endocrine system. Choline has been known to help reduce symptoms of depression, memory loss, and seizures. Endurance athletes also use choline as an aid to build and maintain muscle as well as combat fatigue throughout peak training periods. Choline will methylate estrogen molecules.

Betaine

Estrogen, structurally, is imbalanced. Essentially, the molecule is not structurally complete and requires an extra methyl group for this to occur. Once the estrogen molecule is methylated, it is rendered inert and therefore is pretty useless in the body. The body will then rid itself of the molecule through a process known as chelation.

This is a quite straightforward and effective way of lowering estrogen levels. <u>Betaine and choline are the most effective methylators for estrogen</u>. The best sources of betaine include beets, wheat bran, spinach, and shrimp.

By consuming adequate amounts of an estrogen methylator regularly, you will start to see lower estrogen levels and higher T levels in no time.

Creatine

Creatine monohydrate is a substance produced naturally in the body and aids in the production of another naturally occurring substance known as Adenosine triphosphate (ATP).

ATP provides vital energy during muscle contractions and allows the body to perform short bouts of explosive movements. ATP is what allows a weight lifter to execute those heavy barbell squats and deadlifts.

More creatine means more ATP; more ATP means getting in that extra repetition or two when your body is screaming no mas. This, in turn, translates to optimal muscle stimulation and gains.

In one study, men subjected to rigorous resistance training and administered creatine had higher T levels than from their original baseline. Additionally, they also had higher androgen levels than men who underwent the same training but took a placebo.

In another study conducted in South Africa, rugby players administered 20-grams of creatine monohydrate for seven days saw a 56% increase dihydrotestosterone (DHT) levels.

Testosterone has far stronger androgenic properties when converted into DHT. Once a DHT hormone, it cannot convert into estrogen as is the potential case with regular testosterone.

RESOURCES:

abstract;jsessionid=ACA9D6579BE6093271D030A566E23BA8.f02t04

http://www.jbc.org/content/271/33/19900.short

http://ijrapronline.com/issues3/UK_PATIL_IJRAPR_16-23.pdf

About The Anabolic Men Marketplace

We founded the AM Marketplace upon one simple mission: to provide our readers and customers with a trustworthy one-stop-shop for all of the supplemental needs.

It has become incredibly difficult to sift through all the garbage in the current fitness and supplement industry. Many companies claim to have high quality ingredients when in reality their formulas contain less than 10% of the ingredients actually listed on the bottle.

These practices of cutting corners and screwing the customer while the marketers are in search of making a quick buck has led the supplement industry into a state of ruin and distrust. We opened the AM Marketplace on **store.anabolicmen.com** to provide you with a place where we only stock the highest quality, lab tested, pure ingredients provided by the best brands available.

We source most of our products via a direct partnership with a distribution partner who only sells to physicians & medical professionals, but in our case we worked with them on a solution by providing documentation of professional qualification through Duke University in Durham, North Carolina.

We will never put anything in the AM Marketplace that doesn't have clinical proof of its effectiveness and that isn't from a highly reputable brand. So you can rest assured that since you're part of the Anabolic Men Family, you will be provided with the most effective, highest purity supplemental solutions available.

Go check out the AM Marketplace now at store.anabolicmen.com

Chapter 10

Training Log

Second by second you lose the opportunity to become the person you want to be. Take charge of your life.

— Greg Plitt

I nside this chapter of the program you will find your training log.

This is a blank template you can bring with you to the gym to track your training. Remember, you must always force continual progression, therefore forcing your body into an adaptive state.

Your THOR Log

In this section we encourage you to track your training for your first weeks on the protocol. When you run out of space, you can also download the PDF version of this training log at **anabolicmen.com/ thor-logs** for free, print them out, put them into a binder.

A	B	C	D	E
FOCUS:	SET 1	SET 2	SET 3	SET 4
Date:				
CHECKPOINT LIFT(S)				
ASSISTANCE LIFT(S)				
SPECIALTY LIFT				
NOTES:				

A	B	C	D	E
FOCUS:	SET 1	SET 2	SET 3	SET 4
Date:				
CHECKPOINT LIFT(S)				
ASSISTANCE LIFT(S)				
SPECIALTY LIFT				
NOTES:				

A	B	C	D	E
FOCUS:	**SET 1**	**SET 2**	**SET 3**	**SET 4**
Date:				
CHECKPOINT LIFT(S)				
ASSISTANCE LIFT(S)				
SPECIALTY LIFT				
NOTES:				

A	B	C	D	E
FOCUS:	**SET 1**	**SET 2**	**SET 3**	**SET 4**
Date:				
CHECKPOINT LIFT(S)				
ASSISTANCE LIFT(S)				
SPECIALTY LIFT				
NOTES:				

A	B	C	D	E
FOCUS:	**SET 1**	**SET 2**	**SET 3**	**SET 4**
Date:				
CHECKPOINT LIFT(S)				
ASSISTANCE LIFT(S)				
SPECIALTY LIFT				
NOTES:				

A	B	C	D	E
FOCUS:	**SET 1**	**SET 2**	**SET 3**	**SET 4**
Date:				
CHECKPOINT LIFT(S)				
ASSISTANCE LIFT(S)				
SPECIALTY LIFT				
NOTES:				

A	B	C	D	E
FOCUS:	SET 1	SET 2	SET 3	SET 4
Date:				
CHECKPOINT LIFT(S)				
ASSISTANCE LIFT(S)				
SPECIALTY LIFT				
NOTES:				

A	B	C	D	E
FOCUS:	SET 1	SET 2	SET 3	SET 4
Date:				
CHECKPOINT LIFT(S)				
ASSISTANCE LIFT(S)				
SPECIALTY LIFT				
NOTES:				

A	B	C	D	E
FOCUS:	SET 1	SET 2	SET 3	SET 4
Date:				
CHECKPOINT LIFT(S)				
ASSISTANCE LIFT(S)				
SPECIALTY LIFT				
NOTES:				

A	B	C	D	E
FOCUS:	SET 1	SET 2	SET 3	SET 4
Date:				
CHECKPOINT LIFT(S)				
ASSISTANCE LIFT(S)				
SPECIALTY LIFT				
NOTES:				

Page 140

A	B	C	D	E
FOCUS:	**SET 1**	**SET 2**	**SET 3**	**SET 4**
Date:				
CHECKPOINT LIFT(S)				
ASSISTANCE LIFT(S)				
SPECIALTY LIFT				
NOTES:				

A	B	C	D	E
FOCUS:	**SET 1**	**SET 2**	**SET 3**	**SET 4**
Date:				
CHECKPOINT LIFT(S)				
ASSISTANCE LIFT(S)				
SPECIALTY LIFT				
NOTES:				

A	B	C	D	E
FOCUS:	SET 1	SET 2	SET 3	SET 4
Date:				
CHECKPOINT LIFT(S)				
ASSISTANCE LIFT(S)				
SPECIALTY LIFT				
NOTES:				

A	B	C	D	E
FOCUS:	SET 1	SET 2	SET 3	SET 4
Date:				
CHECKPOINT LIFT(S)				
ASSISTANCE LIFT(S)				
SPECIALTY LIFT				
NOTES:				

A	B	C	D	E
FOCUS:	SET 1	SET 2	SET 3	SET 4
Date:				
CHECKPOINT LIFT(S)				
ASSISTANCE LIFT(S)				
SPECIALTY LIFT				
NOTES:				

A	B	C	D	E
FOCUS:	SET 1	SET 2	SET 3	SET 4
Date:				
CHECKPOINT LIFT(S)				
ASSISTANCE LIFT(S)				
SPECIALTY LIFT				
NOTES:				

A	B	C	D	E
FOCUS:	SET 1	SET 2	SET 3	SET 4
Date:				
CHECKPOINT LIFT(S)				
ASSISTANCE LIFT(S)				
SPECIALTY LIFT				
NOTES:				

A	B	C	D	E
FOCUS:	SET 1	SET 2	SET 3	SET 4
Date:				
CHECKPOINT LIFT(S)				
ASSISTANCE LIFT(S)				
SPECIALTY LIFT				
NOTES:				

A	B	C	D	E
FOCUS:	**SET 1**	**SET 2**	**SET 3**	**SET 4**
Date:				
CHECKPOINT LIFT(S)				
ASSISTANCE LIFT(S)				
SPECIALTY LIFT				
NOTES:				

A	B	C	D	E
FOCUS:	**SET 1**	**SET 2**	**SET 3**	**SET 4**
Date:				
CHECKPOINT LIFT(S)				
ASSISTANCE LIFT(S)				
SPECIALTY LIFT				
NOTES:				

	A	B	C	D	E
		SET 1	SET 2	SET 3	SET 4
FOCUS:					
Date:					
CHECKPOINT LIFT(S)					
ASSISTANCE LIFT(S)					
SPECIALTY LIFT					
NOTES:					

	A	B	C	D	E
		SET 1	SET 2	SET 3	SET 4
FOCUS:					
Date:					
CHECKPOINT LIFT(S)					
ASSISTANCE LIFT(S)					
SPECIALTY LIFT					
NOTES:					

Page 146

A	B	C	D	E
FOCUS:	SET 1	SET 2	SET 3	SET 4
Date:				
CHECKPOINT LIFT(S)				
ASSISTANCE LIFT(S)				
SPECIALTY LIFT				
NOTES:				

A	B	C	D	E
FOCUS:	SET 1	SET 2	SET 3	SET 4
Date:				
CHECKPOINT LIFT(S)				
ASSISTANCE LIFT(S)				
SPECIALTY LIFT				
NOTES:				

A	B	C	D	E
FOCUS:	SET 1	SET 2	SET 3	SET 4
Date:				
CHECKPOINT LIFT(S)				
ASSISTANCE LIFT(S)				
SPECIALTY LIFT				
NOTES:				

A	B	C	D	E
FOCUS:	SET 1	SET 2	SET 3	SET 4
Date:				
CHECKPOINT LIFT(S)				
ASSISTANCE LIFT(S)				
SPECIALTY LIFT				
NOTES:				

A	B	C	D	E
FOCUS:	SET 1	SET 2	SET 3	SET 4
Date:				
CHECKPOINT LIFT(S)				
ASSISTANCE LIFT(S)				
SPECIALTY LIFT				
NOTES:				

A	B	C	D	E
FOCUS:	SET 1	SET 2	SET 3	SET 4
Date:				
CHECKPOINT LIFT(S)				
ASSISTANCE LIFT(S)				
SPECIALTY LIFT				
NOTES:				

A	B	C	D	E
FOCUS:	SET 1	SET 2	SET 3	SET 4
Date:				
CHECKPOINT LIFT(S)				
ASSISTANCE LIFT(S)				
SPECIALTY LIFT				
NOTES:				

A	B	C	D	E
FOCUS:	SET 1	SET 2	SET 3	SET 4
Date:				
CHECKPOINT LIFT(S)				
ASSISTANCE LIFT(S)				
SPECIALTY LIFT				
NOTES:				

A	B	C	D	E
FOCUS:	**SET 1**	**SET 2**	**SET 3**	**SET 4**
Date:				
CHECKPOINT LIFT(S)				
ASSISTANCE LIFT(S)				
SPECIALTY LIFT				
NOTES:				

A	B	C	D	E
FOCUS:	**SET 1**	**SET 2**	**SET 3**	**SET 4**
Date:				
CHECKPOINT LIFT(S)				
ASSISTANCE LIFT(S)				
SPECIALTY LIFT				
NOTES:				

A	B	C	D	E
FOCUS:	SET 1	SET 2	SET 3	SET 4
Date:				
CHECKPOINT LIFT(S)				
ASSISTANCE LIFT(S)				
SPECIALTY LIFT				
NOTES:				

A	B	C	D	E
FOCUS:	SET 1	SET 2	SET 3	SET 4
Date:				
CHECKPOINT LIFT(S)				
ASSISTANCE LIFT(S)				
SPECIALTY LIFT				
NOTES:				

Page 152

A	B	C	D	E
FOCUS:	SET 1	SET 2	SET 3	SET 4
Date:				
CHECKPOINT LIFT(S)				
ASSISTANCE LIFT(S)				
SPECIALTY LIFT				
NOTES:				

A	B	C	D	E
FOCUS:	SET 1	SET 2	SET 3	SET 4
Date:				
CHECKPOINT LIFT(S)				
ASSISTANCE LIFT(S)				
SPECIALTY LIFT				
NOTES:				

What's Next?

Thanks for reading.

We're very glad to have you in the Anabolic Men community. As you train on the THOR Program and use the intelligent supplementation and nutrition advice to naturally optimize your hormones, we want to continue to provide you ample support over on our website **anabolicmen.com**, our YouTube channel, and in the forums.

If you ever need any help or advice on training, nutrition, or supplementation first search the website for information (we've written hundreds upon hundreds of free articles on nearly every subject imaginable so you'll probably find some good info), and if you can't find anything to answer your question, feel free to email our helpful support team at **support@anabolicmen.com**

Welcome to the Family, thank you for your support, and we look forward to hearing your success stories soon and helping you solve all your men's health problems naturally.

-
Chris and Ali

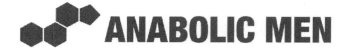 **ANABOLIC MEN**

Made in the USA
San Bernardino, CA
07 June 2017